Federal Priorities in Funding Alcohol and Drug Abuse Programs

Federal Priorities in Funding Alcohol and Drug Abuse Programs

Barry Stimmel, MD, Editor

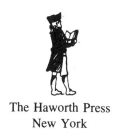

The Haworth Press
New York

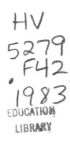
Federal Priorities in Funding Alcohol and Drug Abuse Programs has also been published as *Advances in Alcohol & Substance Abuse,* Volume 2, Number 3, Spring 1983.

The Haworth Press, Inc., 28 East 22 Street, New York, NY 10010

Library of Congress Cataloging in Publication Data
Main entry under title:

Federal priorities in funding alcohol and drug abuse programs.

"Has also been published as Advances in alcohol & substance abuse, volume 2, number 3, spring 1983''—t.p. verso.
Includes bibliographical references.
1. Federal aid to alcoholism programs—United States. 2. Federal aid to drug abuse treatment programs—United States. I. Stimmel, Barry, 1939- . [DNLM: 1. Alcoholism. 2. Financing, Government—United States. 3. Health planning—United States. 4. Research support. 5. Substance abuse. WL AD432 v.2 no.3 / WM 270 F293]
HV5279.F42   1983   362.2'9256'0973   83-6111
ISBN 0-86656-195-1

Federal Priorities in Funding Alcohol and Drug Abuse Programs

Advances in Alcohol & Substance Abuse
Volume 2, Number 3

CONTENTS

EDITORIAL

Federally Sponsored Research: The End of an Era

Society tends to ignore that which it does not wish to see. This approach to the unpleasant encompasses all spheres of life; the medical arena being no exception. While "glamour" diseases, such as coronary artery disease, cancer, and diabetes, are frequently the focus of concern and the recipients of considerable public and private funding, other less socially acceptable conditions, such as alcoholism and substance abuse, are often treated sensationally, too quickly subsiding into newspaper "morgues" until once again resurrected at an appropriate newsworthy time.

It was, therefore, with considerable anticipation that scientists working in the fields of alcoholism and substance abuse observed the formation of the National Institute on Drug Abuse (NIDA) and the National Institute on Alcohol Abuse and Alcoholism (NIAAA) under the auspices of the Alcohol, Drug Abuse, and Mental Health Administration (ADAMHA) in the early 1970s. This elevation to institute status made possible realization by the public of the science involved in the study of alcoholism and substance abuse, as well as a stated commitment by the government to funding similar to that provided to the institutes of the National Institutes of Health (NIH).

To a certain extent these objectives were fulfilled. Both NIDA and NIAAA were sufficiently, if not generously, funded. This allowed the development of a systematic approach to alcohol and substance abuse problems through funding of basic and clinical research, epidemiological studies, evaluation of treatment efficacy and provision of programs to train basic and clinical scientists. The papers in this issue are directed towards assessing the progress that has been made by both institutes, as well as attempting to formulate predictions for the future.

Grupenhoff,[1] from the vantage point of a home base in Washington, attempts to define future congressional support for alcoholism and substance abuse. It is clear that funds to support training grants will no longer be available. This deemphasis in training of qualified personnel is not unique to either NIDA or NIAAA and is occurring throughout all the institutes of the NIH. However, one might argue that this action is less justifiable in the fields of alcoholism and substance abuse. Unfortunately, few professionals are committed to caring for these patients, and the general level of awareness of appropriate management by other physicians is far from optimal. This has resulted in persons drinking excessively escaping early diagnosis and persons abusing drugs being referred to large "drug" centers, thus fostering the concept of alcoholism and substance abuse being "someone else's" problem.

The development and implication of the "block grant mechanism" will also ultimately adversely affect treatment programs. The extent to which programs will feel this pressure is unclear; however, as the economy worsens, states will increasingly attempt to divert funds from treatment in order to meet growing deficits in other areas of concern.

Despite the reorganization that has occurred within both institutes and the commitment of Congress toward continued support of research in alcoholism and substance abuse, these programs must still be considered "endangered species." Most recently, the Office of Management and Budget (OMB) has proposed sweeping changes in the nation's health programs which will include dismantling of the Alcohol, Drug Abuse, and Mental Health Administration and dispersing its functions to other agencies.[2] Although it is quite unlikely that this will occur, nonetheless, the OMB proposal serves as a reminder of the rapid shift in priorities that can occur in response to fiscal imperatives.

Fortunately, the chances of continued research support in both the basic sciences and clinical sciences transiently appear somewhat brighter. Both NIDA and NIAAA have reorganized to meet this challenge and have clearly delineated priority areas.[3-6] It would be well for potential investigators to carefully read the papers addressing these subjects in an attempt to maximize extramural support.

One new major objective that is especially commendable is the rapid dissemination of research results to all persons engaged in the areas of alcoholism and substance abuse. Not infrequently such findings remain unknown to concerned professionals until appearing in journals a year or two subsequent to the completion of a study. The development of any system that would diminish this "lag time" is most certainly welcome.

The review of the actual application process at both institutes, presented for the first time within a single source, allows the reader to determine the specific types of applications that are available.[7] The importance of peer review and the actual mechanism by which a grant is approved are discussed in detail and will be of considerable interest to investigators wishing to pursue extramural support.

Finally, the "Selective Guide" at the end of this issue provides a comprehensive review of existing resources for those who wish to pursue available funding sources. In these times of diminishing resources and elimination of federally supported training grants, the information presented in the guide is particularly relevant.

In summary, although there is certainly not an abundance of Federal support for research and treatment programs in the fields of alcoholism and drug abuse, nonetheless, the maintenance of a commitment on the part of Congress is grounds for cautious optimism. Such support will allow investigators to continue working toward making meaningful contributions. These efforts will, hopefully, be applied clinically to allow for the development of more effective prevention and rehabilitation for those in most need of these services, as well as foster an atmosphere of learning for those professionals committed to the fields of alcoholism and substance abuse.

Barry Stimmel, MD

REFERENCES

1. Grupenhoff JT. Congressional support for alcohol and substance abuse programs: redefining priorities. Advances in Alcohol & Substance Abuse. 1983; 2:5-13.

2. Association of American Medical Colleges: Weekly Report #82-41. December 2, 1982. Washington D.C.

3. Nieberding S. The evolution of the National Institute on Alcohol Abuse and Alcoholism. Advances in Alcohol & Substance Abuse. 1983; 2:15-21.

4. Rosenthal LS. Federal funding of research and research training programs in alcohol abuse: priority areas and mechanisms of support. Advances in Alcohol & Substance Abuse. 1983; 2:23-37.

5. Durell J et al. The National Institute on Drug Abuse: a progress report. Advances in Alcohol & Substance Abuse. 1983; 2:39-47.

6. Durell J et al. The National Institute on Drug Abuse: priorities in funding. Advances in Alcohol & Substance Abuse. 1983; 2:49-58.

7. Durell J et al. The application process at the National Institute on Drug Abuse and the National Institute on Alcohol Abuse and Alcoholism. Advances in Alcohol & Substance Abuse. 1983; 2:59-70.

Congressional Support for Alcohol and Substance Abuse Programs: Redefining Priorities

John T. Grupenhoff, PhD

ABSTRACT. Federal programs and funding patterns for alcohol and substance abuse are in considerable flux at this time. The recent elections for the U.S. Senate and U.S. House of Representatives will have an impact on decisions made as to policy and funding. Also, regulations are now being developed which will change the shape of agencies administering the programs, and such regulations will be impacted seriously by the Budget Reconciliation Act of 1981. These recent events are best understood by reference to funding over the last decade through the Department of Health and Human Services.

INTRODUCTION

Over the last several years, alcohol and substance abuse programs and funding levels in the Federal agencies have been in a state of considerable flux, not unlike the period of the early 1970s during the Nixon Administration, when the attempt was made to alter programmatic efforts, not only by legislation, but also by impoundments of appropriated funds.

This study relates the situation and potential impact of the recent (November, 1982) elections for the U.S. Senate and the U.S. House of Representatives, both in terms of the likely attitudinal changes of the two houses of Congress regarding domestic programs, and of the election's impact upon the authorization and appropriations sub-

Dr. Grupenhoff is a partner in the firm of Grupenhoff and Endicott, Washington, DC, and Lecturer, Department of Health Care Administration, Mount Sinai School of Medicine of the City University of New York.

committees and committees of the Congress which must deal legislatively with these programs. Also, analysis and comment is given on the funding patterns for alcohol and substance abuse programs over the last decade, with some analysis of the FY 1983 appropriations activity in the House and Senate. Finally, some comment will be made about current efforts to modify programs by means of regulations, with top administrators drawing upon authorities granted by the Congress in the 1981 Budget Reconciliation Act.*

IMPACT OF ELECTIONS ON ALCOHOL AND SUBSTANCE ABUSE PROGRAMS

The recent elections resulted in a net increase of 26 Democrats in the U.S. House of Representatives, currently controlled by the Democratic party, and a stand-off in the Senate, now controlled by the Republican party. It is not yet clear how the flavor of the debate will be changed from the last Congress, even though most commentators and observers of Congress indicate that some moderation of efforts of Reagan economics, including less severe cutbacks on domestic programs, will take place. However, the high projected national debt for the next several years will surely prevent any major increase for any of the Federal health and research programs.

Overall election results do not tell the significant story, however. Most major policy issues are fought out in subcommittee and committee, and that is where the Administration and agency and outside interest groups lobby most vigorously. Generally it can be said in health and medicine issues that fully 90% or more of the major decisions on programs and appropriations take place at the subcommittee or committee level, and that the general good or ill will of the Congress as a whole regarding programs is important in terms of providing the climate in which these committees work. Agencies favored by the Congress overall will have little difficulty over their

---

*As this issue goes to press, the President's proposed budget for fiscal year 1984 has just been sent to Capitol Hill, and includes substantial program increases. In Drug Abuse programs, the President proposes a $9.2 million increase in research (19%), an $82,000 increase in training (10%) and a $1 million increase in direct program operations, giving an overall proposed increase of 16.9% for the program. In Alcoholism, research was increased by $12.5 million (37%), training by $115,000 and direct operations by $1.7 million, giving an overall increase of 32% for the program. Also, the President proposed that the ADAMH block grant remain at the fiscal 1983 level of $439 million, and its operations be transferred to the Office of the Assistant Secretary for Health (as are other similar block grant programs).

bills when they come to the Senate or House floor for a full vote, but agencies distrusted or looked at askance by the full Congress are subject to detailed debate and amendment on the floor, regardless of the good will held for them at the committee level. Seasoned observers have long noted that frequently congressional subcommittees and the agencies they deal with legislatively work closely together, and often develop shared attitudes, and when outside interest groups work closely with both in the development of policy, the ties become stronger. Not always, however, are the committee chairman's or the committee's views synchronous with the overall membership of the pertinent full house.

AUTHORIZATION SUBCOMMITTEES AND COMMITTEES AFTER ELECTIONS

In the U.S. House of Representatives, the recent trends are likely to continue, in terms of support for alcoholism and substance abuse programs. It is quite likely that the *authorization* committee of the House, which periodically reauthorizes the legislative authorities under which the programs operate, will be slightly more favorable than before. The full Energy and Commerce Committee, which is the full committee handling the authorizations, will likely add two or perhaps three more Democrats to its majority, and the Republican side will be reduced by that number. The Subcommittee on Health and the Environment, which holds hearings and develops a bill to be sent to the full committee for agreement before it is sent to the floor, also will show a Democratic increase, perhaps one additional member. The significance of these changes, which may seem to be only slight, is in fact considerable. The subcommittee and full committee over the last two years were often deadlocked, with conservative Democrats supporting Republicans on the committee in a number of votes. Thus, with the changes likely to take place, the subcommittee and full committee majorities will likely prevail more often than before.

In the Senate, the situation regarding the authorization is similar to that in the past two years. The chairman and key ranking members of both the majority (Republican) and minority likely will remain the same. Here, too, over the last two years, there were frequent deadlocks, as some moderate Republicans would vote with the Democratic minority to prevent the reporting out of a bill to the floor for full vote. The difficulties faced by the majority, and its staff which does a good deal of negotiating on controversial matters, were considerable this past year. Thus it can be said that generally the pattern here will be the same: a conservative chairman, a supporter of the Administration, will continue to have difficulty pushing forward Administration positions in his committee, and thus in the Senate.

In summary, it can be expected that the House committee and subcommittee will likely be more favorable to authorizations of higher appropriations for alcohol and substance abuse programs, if such legislation comes before them in some fashion. However, it should also be realized that the 1981 Budget Reconciliation Act, which among other things folded the Alcohol Institute's community-based treatment and rehabilitation components into block grants, has largely determined, in terms of authorizations, where the programs like these are headed, and it is to be expected that the Administration will take advantage of the 1981 law to put as many program changes in place as it feels it can by regulation consistent with that law.

APPROPRIATIONS SUBCOMMITTEES AND COMMITTEES

The *appropriations* subcommittees and full committees in both houses provide the funds for the programs authorized by the authorizing committees.

In the House, the Appropriations Committee was changed little by the elections, and the Subcommittee on Labor-HHS, which nearly always produces a bill after long hearings and deliberations which frequently is left untouched by full committee action before the bill goes to the floor, will remain exactly the same in the upcoming Congress as in the last Congress. This committee has always been in the vanguard of support for health care and research programs, and while several modifications to alcohol and substance abuse programs will likely occur (as noted below in the funding analysis) nevertheless it can be said that this subcommittee will provide generally constant support.

The situation in the Senate will be different than it was, however. A conservative chairman of the Senate Labor-HHS Subcommittee lost his re-election race, and the likely successors to him are both more moderate, even tending to liberal on health and research matters, than the previous chairman. In the Senate, more so than the House, the chairman sets the tone of the agenda in subcommittee, and provides the original "mark" for program levels. Therefore, it is quite likely that this subcommittee will be somewhat more supportive in the future of alcohol and substance abuse programs than in the past two years, and will seek less to follow the Administration's proposals.

In summary, the Appropriations Committees are likely to be strong supporters of the alcohol and substance abuse programs. However, it should be understood that they can appropriate only for programs already authorized. These committees also must labor within the bounds set for them by authorization levels, and most importantly by the legislation provided by the 1981 Budget Reconciliation Act.

FUNDING PATTERNS: PAST AND PRESENT

Taking the decade of 1972-1982, the following program and funding trends are noted for both alcohol and drug abuse: research, both intramural and extramural; training, both clinical and research; and service programs. In the case of alcohol programs, some projections can be made about programs from draft documents intended to be presented in regulatory form before the end of 1982, which rely on the 1981 Budget Reconciliation authorities. No such draft proposals have been obtained for drug abuse program regulations.

Some comment is made about the recent actions in the House (which passed the FY 1983 Labor-HHS appropriations bill on December 1, 1982) and in the Senate where the Senate Subcommittee on Labor-HHS Appropriations, and the Senate full Appropriations Committee completed work on the FY 1983 appropriations bill and filed their report in the December 8, 1982 *Congressional Record,* hoping for the bill to be considered on the Senate floor during the "lame-duck" congressional session, due to end late in December, and passed for presidential signature into law.

It is not known at the time of the writing of this article whether the regular appropriations bill will be made law, or whether there will be a "continuing resolution," to continue programs in lieu of a regular bill, or whether such a resolution would mandate a formula of continuing programs "at the lower of the House or Senate levels," a device used in most past "continuing resolutions."

ALCOHOL ABUSE PROGRAMS

Research

The *extramural research program* was at $7.5 million in 1972, and has been increasing since that time generally, to $13.5 million in 1977, and to $18 million in 1982 (there were two years where funding dropped back somewhat, in 1973 and 1981). The House bill for FY 1983 provided a considerable increase for extramural research, and also provided funds to prevent a 10% decrease for indirect costs of research as proposed by the Administration.

In regard to extramural research, the committee stated,

> The balance of the increases for NIAAA . . . are to support an expansion of their extramural research program . . . and to complete the establishment of an alcoholism clinical research program on the NIH campus. With regard to the former, the Committee is aware that this represents a 50% expansion of the NIAAA extramural research program . . . [1]

The *intramural research program* has undergone a similar growth pattern, rising from $407,000 in 1972 to $5 million in 1982. It is significant to note that most of that growth occurred rapidly since 1977, when the intramural program was at a level of $1.5 million. The language of the House bill report referred to above indicates that the intramural program will share somewhat in those increases.

The Senate committee dollar levels are the same as those of the House in this regard.

Training

Research training was at a level of $148,000 in 1972, at $760,000 in 1977, and doubled to $1.1 million in 1982. For FY 1983 the Administration proposed a level of $1.08 million, but the House subcommittee raised their figure to $1.15, slightly above the 1982 level, for FY 1983.

Clinical training has not fared well recently, nor does the near future indicate anything better. Clinical training in 1972 was at a level of $4.7 million, rising to only $6.4 million by 1976, and then dropping to $4.7 million in 1982. It suffered a considerable drop to

$934,000 in FY 1982, and for FY 1983 the Administration proposed that nothing be appropriated for clinical training, and the House agreed with that level, as did the Senate Committee.

Project Grants, Contracts, and Formula Grants

In 1972 this program was at a level of $69 million, and had risen by 1977 to $129 million. It peaked at $133 million in 1980, fell to $90 million in 1981, and was "block granted" by the 1981 Budget Reconciliation Act. As all of alcohol, drug abuse and mental health programs are contained in the block grant, it is not yet known what the block grant funds available for alcoholism will be. (The Senate committee bill report indicates, "For the Alcohol, Drug Abuse and Mental Health Block Grant, the Committee recommends $446,000,000, an increase over the budget request and House allowance of $14,000,000.)

DRUG ABUSE PROGRAMS

Research

The *extramural research program* was at $17 million in 1972, having experienced a major increase from 1971, when it was at $6.6 million. By 1977 it had reached $31 million, from which it rose to $41 million in 1981, and dropped back to $37 million in 1982.

The *intramural research program* was at $9.6 million in 1972, having suffered a drop from the previous year's level of $12.2 million. It then began to suffer a continuous decline, and by 1977 was at a level of $2.5 million. It rose, two years later, to $4.1 million, then dropped back again, and in 1982 was at $3.6 million.

The House FY 1983 bill, noted above, indicates an increase overall for the research program, calling for a level of $47.3 million for both programs, up from $41 million for both the previous year. It is significant that the Administration had requested an increase to $46.3 million. The bill report language states,

> The increase provided over the President's budget is to be used for the restoration of the proposed 10% reduction in the indirect costs of research grants. The increases over 1982 are in support of the expansion of NIDA's extramural research program requested by the President.[2]

It is clear that there has been a renewal of commitment to the extramural research program, inasmuch as even the Administration proposed an increase of $5 million, in a year when so many other domestic programs were cut back.

The Senate bill levels were the same, in this instance, as those in the House bill.

Training

Research training was at a level of $155,000 in 1972, and after a period marked by some declines and advances, rose to $505,000 by 1977. It had doubled by 1981, but by 1982 had fallen back to $914,000 in obligations. The House-passed bill report indicated that the level spent in FY 1982 was $816,000 and the House went along with the Administration's request of $891,000.

Clinical training here, as in the field of alcoholism, did badly. In 1972 it had a level of $9.5 million, and was at just about the same level five years later. The year 1979, however, marked the last level close to that before a significant decline took place in 1980, 1981, and 1982, at levels of $7.8 million, $6.1 million, and $2.6 million, respectively. The House report indicates that the level of no funding proposed by the Administration was agreed to.

The Senate bill on training had the same levels as the House bill.

Project Grants, Contracts and Formula Grants

As was indicated in the section on alcoholism, this program was also "block granted" in the 1981 Budget Reconciliation Act. Undoubtedly there will be some minor increases, but the amount is not yet known, for FY 1983.

SUMMARY

The programs of alcohol and substance abuse within the Department of Health and Human Services have had a mixed history over the years, but until 1980 showed a general increase of funding. The remarkable drop in funding for clinical training in both areas is the clearest trend, although extramural and intramural research continue to receive moderate increases. These two areas have been compared, often, to their counterparts in the National Institutes of

Health, indicated heretofore as having a favored place in Congress' overall attitudes.

The most serious difficulty overall is that which faces all programs which are not entitlements. It is simply that the ballooning Medicare and Medicaid costs are taking away from the discretionary programs in all fields of health, medicine and research.

It is clear that all those having the responsibility for policymaking in this field are acutely aware of this difficulty, whether at the Office of Management and Budget, or in the committees of the Congress dealing with these issues. Whether moderation of the increases for the entitlements will occur, and whether if it does occur more funds will be available for the discretionary programs, is yet to be seen.

REFERENCES

1. Report 97-894, U.S. House of Representatives, 97th Congress, 2d Session, to accompany H.R. 7205, Departments of Labor, Health, and Human Services, and Education, and Related Agencies Appropriation Bill, 1983, p. 64.

2. Ibid, p. 64.

The Evolution of the National Institute on Alcohol Abuse and Alcoholism

Stephen Nieberding

ABSTRACT. The evolution of the National Institute on Alcohol Abuse and Alcoholism is described. In 1969, the alcohol program consisted of a small research and training center in the Division of Special Mental Health Programs of the National Institute of Mental Health. However, new alcohol legislation enacted in the early 1970s soon elevated the program to a National Institute of greater size and diversity. While the emphasis of the new Institute was on State and community-based treatment and prevention activities, the middle and latter part of the 1970s brought a renewed emphasis on alcohol research programs.

I began my Federal service in June 1969, when I became an administrative assistant in the Division of Extramural Research Programs, National Institute of Mental Health (NIMH). At the time, NIMH had recently experienced a major organizational change and was marking its first anniversary under the newly established Health Services and Mental Health Administration (HSMHA). For 20 years before that, NIMH had been an Institute of the National Institutes of Health (NIH), but the passage of Community Mental Health Centers legislation created an NIMH that was quite different from the other NIH Institutes in terms of program composition, and so an agency framework was designed which would be more suitable to its broadened program mission. The new parent agency, the Health Services and Mental Health Administration, did not represent absolute consistency either, since NIMH had become a composite of research, training and services activities, and was being placed with programs which were primarily services in nature. But the organizational change did serve to promote visibility for the new

Mr. Nieberding is Deputy Executive Officer, National Institute on Alcohol Abuse and Alcoholism; Alcohol, Drug Abuse, and Mental Health Administration, Department of Health and Human Services, 5600 Fishers Lane, Rockville, Maryland 20857.

services component, while preserving the stature of NIMH research and training programs.

The three major extramural functions of NIMH were represented in its divisional structure—Division of Extramural Research Programs, Division of Manpower and Training Programs, and Division of Mental Health Services Programs. Each Division administered a broad range of subject areas; the training Division, for example, administered programs in psychiatry, psychology, social work, psychiatric nursing and other areas. Thus, the organizational pattern of NIMH was established according to its three principal functions, within which various disciplines were addressed. However, there was one exception to this rule. A fourth extramural Division, the Division of Special Mental Health Programs, was comprised of a cluster of subject areas which were considered to be in need of a special focus. In 1969, these areas included suicide prevention, metropolitan problems, crime and delinquency, narcotic addiction and alcoholism. There was a separate Center under the Division for each of these subject areas, and each Center administered its own research and training programs. The National Center for the Prevention and Control of Alcoholism funded 68 research grants and 12 training grants and fellowships for a total of $6.4 million in Fiscal Year 1969.

The annual reports and other organizational materials provided a clear presentation of the NIMH organization and of its recent transition to HSMHA. There were, however, other developments rumbling beneath the surface which newcomers could not have discovered by reviewing the orientation materials. On October 15, 1968, President Johnson had signed P.L. 90-574, which contained new provisions for alcoholism prevention and treatment facilities under the Community Mental Health Centers Act. As funding for these new programs began to be included in the NIMH budget submissions, the need for elevating the status of the Alcohol Center became clear. In 1970, the National Center for the Prevention and Control of Alcoholism was redesignated as the Division on Alcohol Abuse and Alcoholism, NIMH, a move designed to provide increased visibility to the program. But even as this was occurring, additional legislation was being considered to elevate the alcohol program to Institute status. Fiscal Year 1971 could best be described as a kaleidoscope of programs, legislation, and organizational changes—a situation in which new events seemed to be developing even before preceding events could be implemented. For example, staffing grants pursuant to the 1968 legislation were first funded in 1971 because the appropriations process had taken that amount of time to make funds available. This occurred, however, months after President Nixon had signed P.L. 91-616, landmark legislation which, among other things, established the National Institute on Alcohol Abuse and Alcoholism and authorized alcohol project grant and formula grant programs. The significant increases for alcohol programs occurred for the first time in 1972, when nearly $70 million was appropriated for the project and formula grant programs, and the total alcohol budget rose to $87.5 million.

At this point, the appropriations process was in line with the legislation; however, the organizational structure of the NIMH was not. The parent organization, NIMH, shared ''Institute'' status with two of its component parts, the National Institute on Drug Abuse and the National Institute on Alcohol Abuse and Alcoholism. Eventually, the present Alcohol, Drug Abuse, and Mental Health Administration (ADAMHA) became the parent organization with three separate Institutes. The National Institute of Mental Health, under ADAMHA, retained its original divisional structure, but two of the original Centers—Alcohol and Narcotic Addiction—were deleted from the Division of Special Mental Health Programs.

Though administratively operational earlier in the 1970s, the Alcohol, Drug Abuse, and Mental Health Administration (ADAMHA) was established by Statute in 1974. Approximately at the same time, the HSMHA of the Public Health Service became three separate agencies—ADAMHA, Health Resources Administration (HRA), and Health Services Administration (HSA).

THE NATIONAL INSTITUTE ON ALCOHOL ABUSE AND ALCOHOLISM

The statutory creation of NIAAA of 1974 indicated Congressional interest in alcoholism treatment, prevention and State-supported activities. By contrast, the more established research and training programs had moved through this transition relatively unaffected—either by change in legislation or appropriations. The NIAAA Division of Research consisted of an intramural effort amounting to less than half a million dollars and a grant program of $8 million. Training, with appropriations of $6.9 million for grants and fellowships, was included as a program component of the new Division of Prevention.

These Congressionally expanded areas of growth were embodied in the NIAAA's Division of Prevention, Division of Special Treatment and Rehabilitation, and Division of State and Community Assistance. Along with training, the Division of Prevention was engaged in a variety of activities designed to stimulate and improve public awareness of the problem of alcoholism, and to explore techniques which could be applied in the communities to bring about a reduction in the problem. Chief among these efforts were the public services and media activities which were given wide exposure during this period, and the National Clearinghouse for Alcohol Information, which had been formerly part of the Mental Health Clearinghouse.

The Division of Special Treatment and Rehabilitation, the largest Division, reflected the great emphasis which was being placed on community-based treatment and early intervention programs. Many of these programs had been tailored to the needs of target population groups, drinking drivers, the employed population, and many others. In Fiscal Year 1974, more than 700 programs were receiving grant support of over $90 million.

The Division of State and Community Assistance was NIAAA's major focal point for involvement in State-based programs and activities. The alcohol State formula grant program provided the means for assuring a focused program effort in every State, and also established a point of contact, a State Alcohol Authority, in each of the States. This latter development facilitated the formation of a Federal-State communication network which could expedite the transfer of ideas and information not only between the Federal Government and the States, but among the States themselves. The legislative amendments of 1976 further emphasized the State roll by establishing for assisting those States which pass legislation decriminalizing public intoxication under the Uniform Alcoholism Intoxication and Treatment Act.

OBJECTIVES AND GOALS

During the early period of its history, NIAAA devised a number of central functions to enhance the effect of its Division programs and to assist the alcohol field in general. One of these was to provide a continuing assessment of the alcohol problem and to detect new trends in drinking behavior which the field could address. The NIAAA set up a system of data collection, survey instruments, and statistical processes as a means of gaining a national perspective on the problem which could be maintained in the years ahead.

Another basic part of the NIAAA mission was to encourage interest and raise public awareness of alcoholism and alcohol-related problems. During the early years, NIAAA formed associations with many groups, including voluntary agencies, youth organizations, business and industry, other Federal agencies and many more, in an effort to multiply the number of sources engaged in alcohol-related work. Publicity campaigns and media activities had been effective in bringing about an improved public awareness about alcoholism, and more of the traditional helping agencies began to step forward and offer their support.

It was also recognized during this period that alcohol treatment needed to increasingly become part of and integrated into more general health services. To accomplish this need, NIAAA became involved in projects to test the feasibility of insurance coverage for alcoholism services, particularly outpatient services, and to elicit the support of public and private carriers. The need for financial support was also the basis for the Institute's efforts to promote accreditation standards for alcohol treatment facilities and certification standards for alcohol personnel, with the hope that these might enable many programs to qualify for reimbursement under existing insurance systems. The constant expansion of the total capacity for dealing with problems of alcohol abuse and alcoholism was part of the NIAAA mission. In fact, each program and activity seemed designed to serve this broader objective in addition to its specified purpose.

By 1975, many of NIAAA's community-based treatment projects were entering their final year of a 3-year approved project period. More than 100 Indian and poverty alcoholism grants had been inherited by the NIAAA with the dismantling of the Office of Economic Opportunity, and these too were in their third year of support. As the budget request was being formulated for 1976, a discussion arose concerning the total length of Federal support which would be given to alcohol treatment projects. The outcome of this discussion was a schedule of declining Federal support over a total 6-year project period. The American Indian programs were considered exempt from this schedule, and subject instead to a plan to transfer them to the Indian Health Service at the end of their sixth year of funding.

Fiscal Year 1976 was the only year in which the program cuts were made based on this new plan. In 1977, the Congress directed NIAAA to continue support for all approved projects. The Congress did not raise objection to the proposal to transfer the American Indian programs to the Indian Health Service, and this part of the plan was implemented from that point forward.

It was also during this period that Congress placed greater emphasis on the NIAAA research program. The 1976 amendments to NIAAA's basic authorizing legislation contained a new Title V for the research program, which had until then cited the Public Health Service Act as its sole governing authority. Title V contained several major changes—(1) it established a separate funding authorization for alcohol research (intramural and research grants and contracts) at $20, $24 and $28 million annually for Fiscal Years 1977 through 1979, and (2) it established the National Alcohol Research Centers program, with a ceiling of $1 million for each Center and a funding authorization of $6 million annually for Fiscal Years 1977 through 1979. With this prospective growth of the research program, NIAAA, in 1977, broadened its organization to include both an Intramural and Extramural Research Division. It was also at this time that NIAAA entered into discussions with NIH concerning patient care space for its future clinical research facility and Congress appropriated $2 million in Fiscal Year 1977 for the National Alcohol Research Centers program. These events, in combination with modest but steady increases for the regular research grant program, laid the groundwork for future growth and development of the NIAAA's research activities.

In fiscal years 1978 and 1979 NIAAA initiated two new State-based programs, the State Voluntary Resource Development Program and the State Manpower Development Program. The stronger focus on the State as an agent to administer Federal funds and programs prompted NIAAA to shift a number of its community-based treatment projects to the States for their direct administration. Also during this time, the Department announced a major new initiative on alcohol abuse and alcoholism and proposed increases in support of these initiatives, particularly in the areas of research and prevention. NIAAA became deeply involved in the development of a major media campaign directed toward women, young people and mothers of child-bearing age.

The decade of the 1980s brought yet other changes for the alcohol field—namely, the establishment of the alcohol, drug abuse and mental health services block grant. With the clear statutory direction for States to become the focal point for provision of alcoholism prevention and treatment, the role of the Institute also changed. The budget now requests funds for research into alcoholism, alcohol and medical disorders, alcohol-related deaths and injuries, prevention, and epidemiology, as well as support for general public information activities and technical assistance.

Clearly, the decade of the 1980s holds promise for those concerned about alcoholism and alcohol abuse. The federal Government will be directing its efforts to National leadership—including research and technical assistance. States will be coordinating, directing and providing prevention and treatment services tailored to their local needs and priorities. Private health insurors are becoming increasingly interested in utilization and costs—both for an individual and other family members—when they offer in their basic coverage reimbursement for alcoholism treatment. Labor and Management have recognized the gains in productivity achieved by offering employees assistance programs (EAPs). Health care professionals—through basic and continuing education—are becoming increasingly sensitized to alcoholism and alcohol abuse. And Voluntary associations and concerned citizens are making significant impact in heightening public awareness and taking action to prevent alcoholism and alcohol-related problems.

Federal Funding of Research and Research Training Programs in Alcohol Abuse: Priority Areas and Mechanisms of Support

Laura S. Rosenthal

ABSTRACT. To address successfully the breadth and complexity of problems associated with the harmful use of alcohol, the National Institute on Alcohol Abuse and Alcoholism (NIAAA) supports a program of basic and applied research on the causes, processes, and consequences of alcoholism and other alcohol-related problems and on techniques for their detection, prevention, and treatment. Scientific studies in these areas are supported by the NIAAA through several mechanisms. These are discussed as are future program directions and the current areas of research encouraged and supported by the Institute. In addition to research, the NIAAA also supports programs of research training at the predoctoral and postdoctoral levels. The mechanisms of support for these programs, current areas of support, and future directions are also discussed.

A. BACKGROUND

The breadth of health and social problems that have been found to be associated with the harmful use of alcohol requires a research program of parallel scope and complexity. To deal successfully with the difficulties inherent in the treatment and prevention of alcohol-related problems, the National Institute on Alcohol Abuse and Alcoholism (NIAAA) supports a program of scientific studies that addresses itself to the disease of alcoholism as well as to the broad range of alcohol-related problems, including fetal defects, cirrhosis,

Ms. Rosenthal is Former Deputy Associate Director for Research, and is currently Deputy Director, Division of Intramural Clinical and Biological Research, at the National Institute on Alcohol Abuse and Alcoholism, 5600 Fishers Lane, Rockville, MD 20857.

alcoholic cardiomyopathy and other cardiovascular disorders, cancer, pancreatitis, gastritis, Wernicke-Korsakoff's Syndrome, depression, malnutrition, impaired adolescent developmental processes, highway fatalities, child and spouse abuse, aggressive and criminal behaviors, and disrupted family life. In this context, the Institute has conceptualized the research program in terms of two long-range goals: the development of new knowledge so as to reduce the incidence and prevalence of alcohol abuse and alcoholism, and the development of new knowledge to reduce the morbidity and mortality associated with alcohol use, alcohol abuse, and alcoholism. Research in support of these goals is carried out through two primary mechanisms, the extramural support of regular and center grants and contracts, and the direct conduct of scientific studies by the NIAAA through its intramural research effort.

The long-range plan of the NIAAA research efforts is based on the acknowledgement that there is a need to *develop a national research capacity* for the investigation of alcohol-related problems. This situation is unlike that of many other health fields which are already more fully developed and which are now seeking, essentially, to maintain an existing capacity. A national alcohol research program must include the development of institutional research capability as well as of individual investigator competence, and must involve increased training capacity as well as efforts to retain those high-quality scientists already working in the alcohol field and to attract both young investigators and already-established scientists now working in other fields. It is well-recognized that in the development of a high-quality national program, there must be a coordinated agenda of plans and activities to stimulate the field and to direct the growth of the research capacity in an orderly way. The availability of funds per se is not sufficient, although the stimulation of the field without sufficient monies to follow through would serve only to destroy credibility and further inhibit the field's development.

In addition to sufficient funds, of course, there must also be productive areas of scientific opportunity and an interest and ability in the field to pursue these issues. At the request of the NIAAA, the Institute of Medicine/National Academy of Sciences recently undertook an extensive scientific review of the alcohol field for the purpose of identifying more specifically those areas which present the greatest opportunities for productive and useful research. The report concluded that significant research opportunities exist and await investigation in the biomedical, psychosocial, and behavioral areas, and that increased efforts and investments would have significant yields.[1] To support activities in these areas, the NIAAA employs several mechanisms that together function in a coordinated, symbiotic fashion: an extramural regular grant program serves to support the depth and complexity of alcoholism research required on a national level; the centers program adds a multidisciplinary aspect to this research; and the intramural program takes advantage of the unique community of resources available at the National Institutes of Health. In addition, the research centers program and the intramural program serve as training grounds for alcohol researchers, thereby working together with NIAAA-supported research training programs to ensure an adequate supply of investigators as the research effort expands.

B. RESEARCH

1. Program Aims and Future Directions

In keeping with its mission, the NIAAA supports basic and applied research on the causes, processes, and consequences of alcoholism and other alcohol-related problems, and on the critical factors and improved methodology for their identification, prevention, and treatment. Research activities in these areas are funded through several types of grant and contract support, including regular project grants, center grants, small grants, and research scientist development awards (each discussed more fully below). To assist the Institute in planning and monitoring the research program, and communicating its interests to potential investigators, the areas of research supported by the Institute have been conceptualized into six specific program categories: the causes (etiology) of alcohol-related problems; the mechanisms (pathogenesis) by which alcohol exerts its harmful effects and alcohol-related problems develop; the diagnosis and early identification of alcohol-related problems; the development and assessment of improved techniques for the treatment of alcohol-related disorders; the development and assessment of techniques for the prevention of alcohol-related problems; and the development of basic tools and methodologies that will aid in understanding various aspects of these problems. (Each of these areas is discussed in greater detail below.)

While recognizing the interrelated nature of these research categories, the Institute hopes to shift the emphasis of the research program by gradually shifting the percentage distribution of funds among categories. Well over 50 percent of research dollars are now spent on studies concerned with the etiology and pathogenesis of alcohol effects. At the current time, this is appropriate, since at present the largest component of research applications and of high-quality approved-but-unfunded applications are in the areas of etiology and pathogenesis. Depending upon the amount of funds available, it is hoped to gradually decrease this percentage and concomitantly increase the percentage of funds going into the areas of early identification and diagnosis, treatment research, and prevention research. Efforts by Institute staff and increased interest in the research field within the last few years have resulted in an increased level of support in the area of treatment research. Similar increases are desired in the areas of early identification and diagnosis and prevention research, especially. If successful, this shift would mean a more uniform distribution of funds between the areas of etiology and pathogenesis and the areas of treatment, early identification, and prevention research. Such shifts, however, which might improve the programmatic balance of the research effort, must be implemented carefully so as to ensure that the quality of work being supported is not adversely affected, for the quality as well as the relevance of the research produced are the most important determinants of the potential impact of the research and the most important measures of our success.

2. *Areas of Interest - Program Categories*

The major objectives or areas of research encouraged and supported by the Institute are as follows:

a. Etiology. NIAAA supports research on the biomedical, biobehavioral, and psychosocial factors that can function as antecedents of alcoholism and alcohol-related disorders. Research is encouraged to identify and assess the related contributions of genetic and environmental influences, including studies of twins, adoptees, and half-siblings; the determination of environmental factors (including familial, social, cultural, occupational, and personality factors, that may act to predispose or precipitate the development of alcohol problems, and how they may act for specific population subgroups; the identification of contextual and situational variables that can act to facilitate or inhibit drinking behaviors; gender differences in alcohol susceptibility; various physiological and biochemical traits that differ among specific subpopulations; metabolic pathway(s) of alcohol, especially the physiological significance of alcohol dehydrogenase (and its isozymes), catalase, and the microsomal ethanol oxidizing system (MEOS); animal models to assess metabolism; genetic markers; and heightened or diminished inheritable sensitivity to the various pathological conditions including liver diseases, cardiovascular diseases, neutopathology and psychopathology that result from harmful alcohol use.

b. Pathogenesis. NIAAA supports research that specifies the actions of alcohol on the body and the mechanisms by which it exerts its effects. Studies in the following areas are encouraged: the processes of dependence, tolerance, and withdrawal; the effects of alcohol on the physiological properties of cell membrane; the impact of alcohol on central nervous system, neurotransmitters and their receptors; the impact of alcohol use on the fetus, specifically, the potential for behavioral teratogenesis, mechanism(s) for teratogenic action, and identification of critical period(s); the actions of alcohol on peripheral organs, specifically, the development of alcoholic liver disease, alcoholic myopathy and cardiomyopathy, alcohol-related cancer, and interaction between alcohol and coronary artery disease; the effect of alcohol on neuropsychological functioning, cognitive and memory processes, and sensory-motor functions; the impact of alcohol on metabolism, immunological responses, endocrine functions, nutrition, and neuropsychiatric processes; individual and subpopulation differences in metabolic rates and pathways, and the relevance of these differences to the prevalence of alcohol-derived problems and differential organ pathology; the behavioral and physiological mechanisms by which alcohol contributes to disruptive family functioning, impaired adolescent development, abusive and violent behavior, or accidents; interactions of alcohol with other drugs; animal models to assess alcohol intoxication, tolerance, dependence, and toxicity; and the examination of factors in the natural history of alcohol use that ameliorate or exacerbate alcohol problems.

c. Early Identification and Diagnosis. NIAAA encourages research for the development of techniques and procedures to facilitate the early identification and diagnosis of alcohol abusers and of the problems related to alcohol use. This includes the development of laboratory and functional criteria and measures for recognizing the medical and psychosocial complications of alcohol use, as well as the identification and diagnostic assessment of alcohol abusers and individuals at high risk, particularly among special population groups (e.g., women, youth). Relevant techniques involving biochemical, physiological, behavioral, or cognitive measures as well as family history studies are needed.

d. Treatment. NIAAA supports research for the development and assessment of effective treatments for alcoholism and alcohol-related disorders. Studies in the following areas are needed: the development of enhanced methodologies to measure the efficacy of specific treatment modalities and procedures such as detoxification, emergency medical procedures, psychopharmacological therapies, and various types of psychotherapeutic approaches (including, e.g. family or couples therapy); preclinical and clinical studies and clinical trials for the development and assessment of improved therapeutic techniques; the delineation of clinically-relevant diagnostic categories and outcome criteria and improved methods for their measurement; assessment of access to treatment and the factors that contribute to or inhibit the decision to enter care; and studies of untreated alcoholics, the natural history of alcoholism, and the treatment needs of particular subpopulation groups.

e. Prevention. NIAAA encourages research that focuses on the development and identification of fundamental prevention techniques and approaches and that can provide a basis for the subsequent development and evaluation of prevention services programs. Studies in the following areas are supported: the development of enhanced methodologies to measure the efficacy of specific approaches for the prevention of particular alcohol problems; the development of techniques that can be usefully applied in reducing alcohol-related driving and other accidents; the identification of basic principles of learning and motivation as they may apply to alcohol consumption behaviors and to particular alcohol-related problems (e.g., accidents, crimes, family violence); investigation of cultural beliefs, familial influence, peer pressure, occupational factors and employee programs, and advertising as mechanisms which influence or inhibit development of abusive drinking practices and associated behaviors; potential uses of reinforcement or biofeedback techniques to modify alcohol consumption behaviors; the relationship of alcohol consumption levels, patterns, and adverse consequences to alcohol availability and legal or economic sanctions; the relationship of physical setting and social situation to consumption practices; and the development of pharmacologic agents which may counter effects of intoxication or toxic actions of alcohol through enhancement of alcohol elimination rates and other means.

f. Basic Tools and Methodologies. NIAAA encourages research that develops and refines the basic tools and methodologies for use in addressing specific research problems. Support will be provided for the development of animal strains that react in specific and predictable ways to alcohol; the development of techniques for long-term alcohol administration, allowing the study of tolerance and dependence; and the development of animal models for genetic studies and for investigating fetal alcohol effects.

3. Mechanisms of Support

Research is supported by the Institute through several mechanisms. The major types of funding support are described in Program Announcements and Guidelines that are published by the Institute and mailed to universities, medical schools, and professional and other interested associations, and are also available to any interested individual upon request from the Institute. These Guidelines detail areas in which the Institute is interested in receiving applications for funding (described in general above), the application process, and the types of activities and costs which are allowable and for which funding can be provided. This information is summarized as follows:

a. Regular Research Grants. Regular research grants constitute the traditional mechanism available for funding investigator-initiated research projects. All areas of investigation that are clearly related to the etiology, prevalence, prediction, diagnosis, clinical course, treatment, management, or prevention of alcoholism or other alcohol-related health problems, or to consequences of these health problems, are eligible for support under this grant mechanism. As with all research grant support, regular grants are awarded by the Institute following a review of the submitted application by a group of primarily non-Federal scientific experts who evaluate the proposal for its scientific and technical merit, and upon the recommendation of the National Advisory Council on Alcohol Abuse and Alcoholism. Funding decisions are made by the Institute on the basis of the overall scientific and technical merit of the proposal, Institute program balance and relevance of the proposal to NIAAA program objectives, and the availability of funds. Approximately nine months are required for the review and funding process.

Applicants may request funding support for a period of up to 5 years, although the usual length of each grant award tends to be for 3-year periods. Subsequent grant awards may be made by the Institute if requested by the applicant to continue the project; these competing continuation (renewal) awards are subject to the same review procedures as for new grant awards, and must compete successfully for support with other applicants for regular grant funds.

b. Small Grants. The Small Grant Program is intended to provide support for newer, less experienced investigators, investigators at small colleges, and others who do not have regular research grant support or resources available from their institutions for research exploration. Small Grants may be used for exploratory or pilot studies, to develop or test a new technique, or to analyze previously-collected data; support is not provided for dissertation research.

Support under the Small Grant Program is limited to a one-year period and is not renewable. The Program provides up to $14,000 in direct costs for research, as well as indirect costs. Funding is provided by the NIAAA for applications in any scientific area relevant to the mission of the Institute. Small Grants are reviewed by a special initial review group (which is coordinated for the Agency by the National Institute of Mental Health) for scientific merit and by the NIAAA National Advisory Council. Applications are received on a continuous basis and the review process, although similar to that for regular research grants, is considerably faster. Since a primary intent of this program is to encourage new investigators in the alcohol field, the Institute places a high priority on funding approved applications in this category.

c. Research Scientist Development and Research Scientist Awards. Research Scientist Development and Research Scientist Awards are made to investigators who have demonstrated unusual potential or productivity, to enable them to be relieved of their academic responsibilities so that they can devote their full time to the development of their research capabilities, with the goal of raising the level of competence and increasing the number of individuals engaged in particular areas of research. Awards made to talented investigators are intended to promote their long-term work in alcohol research and to assist recipient institutions in establishing or expanding research programs in alcohol-relevant areas.

Several types of awards are available. Research Scientist Development Awards (RSDA) Level I are intended to assist individuals with exceptional research potential who need further supervised research experience. Applicants include well-trained clinicians who desire to pursue a research career, or scientists who wish extensive supervised experience in an additional scientific discipline. Level II awards are designed to support well-trained scientists who are capable of conducting excellent independent research but who need additional research experience to realize their full scientific potential. Level I and II awards are both made for five-year periods of support. Level I awards may not be renewed; Level II awards may be renewed once; total support for Levels I and II may not exceed 10 years. Applicants for both awards must have at least three years of postdoctoral experience.

Research Scientist Awards are intended to support exceptional senior investigators in essentially full-time research positions at departments or centers where institutional funds are not available to support such full-time research activities. These awards, which are made very rarely by the Institute, are intended for those outstanding senior scientists who have made and are likely to continue to make significant contributions to the alcohol field. Awards are made for five-year periods of support and are renewable subject to a highly rigorous and competitive review.

Research Scientist Development Awards and Research Scientist Awards are reviewed through the same dual review process as applies for regular research grants, and likewise require nine months from the submission of an application to award of a grant. Funding decisions are made by the Institute on the basis of overall scientific merit of the proposal, relevance of the proposal to NIAAA program objectives and programmatic balance, and availability of funds. Specific review criteria and terms and conditions that apply to the different types of awards are outlined in the Program Announcement and Guidelines.

d. National Alcohol Research Centers. The National Alcohol Research Centers were initiated in FY 1977 in response to a legislative amendment, and now comprise nine Centers. Consistent with legislative intent, the Centers program is designed to complement the regular research grant program of the Institute by providing long-term support for multidisciplinary research programs that focus on a particular research theme relating to alcoholism and other alcohol-related problems. As with regular research grants, center grants are reviewed through the dual review process, i.e., review by a group of primarily non-Federal scientific experts who evaluate the scientific and technical merit of proposals and by the NIAAA National Advisory Council. Applications recommended for approval by the National Council are considered for funding by the Institute on the basis of overall scientific and technical merit of the proposal, relevance of proposals to the objectives of the Institute and programmatic balance, and the availability of funds. Center grants are funded for project periods up to five years; subsequent renewal support is available contingent on the same review procedures and successful competition with other applicants for center grant support.

e. Contracts. Contracts are used by the Institute on an infrequent basis to support certain research-related activities that are of direct benefit to the Institute and for which a well-defined product or service can be specified in advance. On these occasions, the Institute publishes a special Request for Proposals advertising the contract availability and providing all necessary details.

C. RESEARCH TRAINING

1. Program Aims and Future Directions

The research training program of the NIAAA, known as the National Research Service Award (NRSA) program, is designed to reflect priorities which stem from the needs of the research effort itself. As new knowledge concerning important factors in alcoholism emerges, the NIAAA research training program aims to give priority to these developing research areas. In addition, the Institute views the research training program as a mechanism for encouraging research in particular areas of interest which do not yet have an adequate pool of technically trained investigators, such as the field of clinical research. Since the development of new researchers through training can require up to five years lead time, an investment in research training is an investment directed towards future research progress. A well-balanced research training program should therefore include training directed towards well-recognized aspects of alcohol-derived problems, such as the continuing important problem of alcoholic liver cirrhosis, as well as newly developing areas such as the genetics of alcoholism.

Consistent with the legislation authorizing the NRSA program, an assessment of the role and need for Federal training programs in the biomedical and behavioral sciences is performed each year for the Alcohol, Drug Abuse, and Mental Health Administration and the

National Institutes of Health by the Committee on a Study of National Needs for Biomedical and Behavioral Research Personnel, of the National Academy of Sciences. In keeping with their findings of a potential oversupply of behavioral scientists, the Institute is placing an emphasis on postdoctoral rather than predoctoral support in the behavioral sciences. (This emphasis does not apply to support in other areas of science.)

While recognizing the need for research training support in a broad range of areas, the Institute is also interested in increasing its emphasis on clinical research training, so as to move consistently with and to strengthen the growing research interest in this area. Similarly, the Institute is interested in strengthening its program of support for epidemiologic research training so as to strengthen prevention research programs and the ability to target intervention efforts on particular problems in particularly susceptible groups.

In addition to these areas, the Institute will continue to give emphasis to research training on minority issues relevant to alcohol problems and to the development of minority researchers.

2. Areas of Support

The NIAAA supports research training related to the problems of alcoholism and alcohol use, including alcohol-derived medical and psychosocial problems. Applications for research training are encouraged in the etiology, pathogenesis, diagnosis, treatment, epidemiology, and prevention of alcoholism and other alcohol-related problems. Specific foci of the program are as follows:

a. Basic Studies. Research training is aimed at developing methodologies for understanding the mechanisms of ethanol action on biological and behavioral processes. This includes training in the development of tools and techniques for use in addressing specific research problems, such as the development of animal models for studying the genetic basis of alcoholism and the mechanisms of addiction and intoxication.

b. Incidence and Prevalence (Epidemiology). Trained investigators are needed for epidemiologic research on rates of occurrence and distribution of alcohol use and alcohol-derived problems; understanding of factors involved in differential distribution; and methodologic research involving statistical, interview, and case finding techniques.

c. Etiology, Description, Diagnosis, and Pathogenesis. Research training is supported for the preparation of scientists to conduct studies of biochemical, genetic, psychological, and environmental risk factors in predisposition to alcoholism and alcohol-derived medical consequences; methods for early identification and detection; methods for differential diagnosis; biological and behavioral manifestations and consequences of alcohol-related problems; stages and sequences in alcoholism and research on mechanisms of action of alcohol and the pathological effects on biological and behavioral processes.

d. Treatment Development, Assessment, and Evaluation. Research training is encouraged for the development of investigators to conduct studies aimed at understanding the treatment process, utilizing behavioral, psychosocial, or biomedical techniques; the development of new therapeutic techniques for alcoholism or alcohol-derived disorders; explaining different responses to and outcomes of specific treatment techniques; assessing the safety and efficacy of particular treatments; and improving instruments for measuring treatment outcome.

e. Public Health/Prevention. Support is provided to train investigators for research on factors involved in the utilization, effectiveness, and cost of services; and the effectiveness of prevention intervention approaches, such as early identification, counseling, education/information, and community intervention.

3. Mechanisms of Support

a. NRSA Individual Fellowships. The NIAAA supports National Research Service Awards to individuals for research training in biomedical and behavioral research areas related to alcoholism and alcohol-derived problems. Fellowships are provided at both the predoctoral and postdoctoral levels. Predoctoral applicants must have completed two or more years of graduate work and be enrolled in a doctoral degree program. Applicants for support at the postdoctoral level must have received a professional doctoral degree; awards are not made for study leading to professional degrees. Prior to formal submission of an Award proposal, an applicant must arrange for appointment to an appropriate institution (including ADAMHA or NIH) and acceptance by a sponsor who will supervise the research training. Fellowship support, at either the pre- or postdoctoral level, is limited by Agency policy to three years. Consistent with legislation requirements, recipients of Awards are required, within two years of completion of support, to engage in continuous, health-related, biomedical or behavioral research or teaching for a period of time equal to twelve months less than the period of research training support.

NRSA Fellowship Awards provide limited stipend support to help provide for living expenses during the period of training. Predoctoral support is $5,040; postdoctoral stipends range from $13,380 to $18,780, depending on the number of years of prior relevant postdoctoral experience. Limited institutional allowances ($3,000 for predoctoral and for postdoctoral fellows) are also provided to help defray tuition and fees, research supplies, and related items.

Applications for NRSA Fellowships are reviewed by groups of primarily non-Federal experts for their scientific/educational merit. Funding decisions are made by the Institute on the basis of overall scientific/educational merit, relevance to Institute program objectives, and availability of funds. Approximately seven months are required for the review and award process.

b. NRSA Institutional Awards. National Research Service Awards are provided to institutions to develop or enhance research training opportunities for individuals selected by them for training in careers in alcohol-related biomedical or behavioral research. Support is provided to institutions for research training at the predoctoral or postdoctoral levels. Individuals selected by the institution to receive support at the predoctoral level must have received an appropriate baccalaureate degree and be enrolled in a doctoral degree program; selected postdoctoral trainees must have received a professional doctoral degree (e.g., MD, PhD, ScD); awards are not made for study leading to the professional degree.

Awards for institutional grants are provided for project periods of up to five years. By law, individuals may not receive more than 5 years of support at the predoctoral level and 3 years of support at the postdoctoral level (through an individual fellowship and/or institutional award). Legal requirements for payback service in health-related research or training also apply to trainees supported under NRSA Institutional Grants.

As with Individual Fellowships, stipend support is provided through Institutional Awards to help provide for the trainee's living expenses during the training period. Support at the predoctoral level is $5,040; support at the postdoctoral level ranges from $13,380 to $18,780, depending on the number of years of prior relevant postdoctoral experience. Institutions may also request limited support to help defray tuition and fees; indirect costs (or 8% of allowable direct costs); and currently $1,500 for predoctoral and $2,500 for postdoctoral trainees for research supplies, salaries, and related expenses.

Applications for institutional grants are reviewed by groups of primarily non-Federal experts for their scientific/educational merit, and by the NIAAA National Advisory Council. Applications recommended for approval by the Council are selected for funding by the Institute on the basis of overall scientific/educational merit, emphasis on postdoctoral support if in the behavioral sciences, relevance to Institute programmatic objectives, and availability of funds. Approximately nine months is required from the submission of an application to the earliest possible start date of the Award.

c. ADAMHA Minority Access to Research Careers (MARC) Program. Participation in the ADAMHA MARC Program is one vehicle by which the Institute aims to increase support for the development of minority researchers and for research training in areas relevant to minority issues in alcoholism. The intent of this mechanism is to increase the participation in alcohol-related biomedical and behavioral research of educational institutions with a substantial minority enrollment.

Two types of Awards are available under this program. The Honors Undergraduate Research Training Grants Program is designed to train highly-selected undergraduate students during their third and fourth undergraduate years. Faculty Fellowship Awards are also available for the purpose of strengthening the research capability of the faculty at predominantly minority institutions.

D. APPLICANT ASSISTANCE

Potential applicants for research grants or research training awards are referred to the Program Announcements and Guidelines listed below for more detailed information about available funding support and requirements. Applicants are also encouraged to contact staff of the Institute for grant information and technical assistance in the submission of an application. Program Announcements and Guidelines are available for the following Research and Research Training Programs of the NIAAA:

1. Alcohol Research Grants

2. Alcohol Research Center Grants
3. Small Grants Program
4. Research Scientist Development and Research Scientist Awards
5. National Research Service Awards (Individual and Institutional)
6. ADAMHA Minority Access to Research Careers (MARC): Honors Undergraduate Research Training Grants and Faculty Fellowships

Information may be obtained from the Division of Extramural Research, National Institute on Alchohol Abuse and Alcoholism, 5600 Fishers Lane, Rockville, Maryland 20857 (telephone: 301/443-2530).

REFERENCE

1. *Report of a Study—Alcoholism and Related Problems: Opportunities for Research.* Institute of Medicine/National Academy of Sciences, July 1980.

The National Institute on Drug Abuse: A Progress Report

Jack Durell, MD, and the Staff
at the National Institute
on Drug Abuse

ABSTRACT. The National Institute on Drug Abuse (NIDA) was established in 1973 as the lead Federal agency for drug abuse education, training, treatment, rehabilitation, and research. Working with designated Single State Agencies (SSAs), NIDA developed an effective and flexible Federal-State partnership, with SSAs given increasing responsibility for planning and administering drug abuse prevention and treatment services within their States.

Since the advent of the Alcohol, Drug Abuse, and Mental Health Services Block Grant Program in FY 1982, NIDA no longer provides direct financial assistance to treatment and prevention program. Instead, it is being organized into function units in: general areas of basic biological studies of drug and substance abuse; animal and human studies revelant to developing more effective treatment and prevention activities; and epidemiological studies. Another important unit will disseminate research findings and other relevant information to researchers, clinicians, and the public.

NIDA's research program has made several major contributions in the past several years. These include: (1) the identification and isolation of opiate receptors and of endogenous opiate-like substances; (2) the development of techniques for swiftly and reliably assessing drug abuse trends and of ongoing epidemiological data systems; (3) the development of new and more effective drug abuse treatment agents, most notably LAAM, naltrexone, and buprenorphine; (4) the classification of the addictive properties of nicotine; (5) the controlled testing of several school-based drug abuse prevention strategies; (6) the completion of a unique study on the drug paraphernalia market; (7) a large-scale investigation of drug use patterns in rural areas; (8) important data on what types of treatment are most effective for particular types of drug abusers.

Dr. Durell is Associate Director for Science, National Institute on Drug Abuse, 5600 Fishers Lane, Rockville, Maryland 20857.

HISTORY

By the late 1960s there was a high level of concern over increasing use of illegal psychoactive drugs in the United States and widespread pressure from many sides for the Federal government to become involved in attacking the problem. The establishment of the Special Action Office for Drug Abuse Prevention (SAODAP) in June 1971 marked the beginning of a coordinated Federal drug abuse prevention effort centralized in the White House. The office identified the need for a comprehensive program which would incorporate drug abuse education, training, treatment, rehabilitation, and research. This resulted in the passage of the "Drug Abuse Office and Treatment Act of 1972" (PL 92-255), which officially established SAODAP for a three-year period and provided funds to support existing programs or new programs implemented by that office. The Act also established the framework for a nationwide system of drug abuse prevention, treatment, and rehabilitation projects in which Federal, State, and local agencies would bear clearly defined responsibilities for carrying out these national goals. Finally, this Act also called for the establishment of the National Institute on Drug Abuse in the Department of Health, Education and Welfare, to continue the work of SAODAP after its term expired in June 1975.

As a result of that Act and of the Reorganization Order of the Secretary of the Department of Health, Education and Welfare, the National Institute on Drug Abuse (NIDA) was established on September 25, 1973. It brought together into one place a number of already operative Federal drug abuse program initiatives, primarily from the National Institute of Mental Health (NIMH) and the Special Action Office for Drug Abuse Prevention. The Reorganization Order which established NIDA was subsequently incorporated into legislation, the "Comprehensive Alcohol Abuse and Alcohol Prevention, Treatment, and Rehabilitation Act Amendments of 1974" (PL 93-282, Section 204).

Believing that program management should be undertaken by those officials closest to actual service delivery, the Department, and within it NIDA, worked on developing an effective and flexible Federal-State partnership. Under this system specially designated Single State Agencies for Drug Abuse (SSAs) were given responsibility for managing treatment, prevention, and training resources. The Federal government also looked to the SSAs to develop State-level standards of care, training programs, and funding sources, while it provided policy guidance, consultation, and technical assistance. With the development of Federal strategies and policies, more and more responsibility for planning and administering drug abuse treatment services within States went to the Single State Agencies (SSAs) within each State. In fact, in the past several years the SSAs have become the primary planners, coordinators, and administrators of drug abuse treatment and prevention services within their respective States.

Until fiscal year 1982, the Statewide Services Grant Program and the Formula Grant Program, authorized under Sections 410 and 409 of Public Law 92-255, as amended, were the primary mechanisms through which treatment and prevention services were funded. The Statewide Services Grant was funded on a cost-sharing, cost-reimbursement basis. The SSA had the responsibility for the administration, coordination and monitoring of the treatment programs under the grant. This allowed for federally supported treatment services to be delivered within a State under the authority of the State agency responsible for drug abuse planning and coordination. This mechanism also provided the SSAs with considerable flexibility in the management and administration of drug abuse treatment services within their States.

A second funding mechanism, known as the State Drug Abuse Formula Grant Program, allowed financial assistance to be provided to the States for planning, establishing, conducting and coordinating projects for the development of more effective drug abuse prevention functions in the State and for evaluating the conduct of such functions.

The ending of the fiscal year 1981 marked the beginning of a new Federal effort, the Alcohol and Drug Abuse and Mental Health Services (ADMS) Block Grant Program. This program replaced both the Statewide Services Grant Program and the Formula Grant Program. The advent of the new ADMS Block Grant meant that the States officially undertook full responsibility for many functions which they already were carrying out. Although it no longer provides direct financial assistance to treatment and prevention programs, NIDA continues to carry on a number of important activities which have a direct bearing on these programs' effective operations.

MISSION AND STRUCTURE

Until recently NIDA's research program was carried out within the context of an organization structure that primarily involved two divisions: the Division of Research and the Division of Resource Development. Within these divisions six major areas were addressed: (1) research; (2) prevention; (3) treatment; (4) training; (5) information development and dissemination; and (6) international drug abuse control. Following the decision to place more emphasis and importance on the development of new and more effective treatment and prevention techniques, the structure of the Division of Resource Development was modified and its name changed to the Division of Treatment and Prevention Development. In addition to emphasizing certain areas of research, the purpose of this change was to attempt to develop an administrative structure that would facilitate the movement of findings from the basic research program through clinical trials and to clinical practice.

Once the decision was made to fund State drug abuse programs through the block grant mechanism in 1981, the functions of NIDA were further refined to focus on research and the dissemination of its findings for a variety of purposes, including: (1) prevention activities; (2) treatment strategies; and (3) increasing the knowledge base. Starting from this goal NIDA has developed a reorganization plan, the final details of which are currently under review.

The basic philosophy of the plan, however, is to create separate functional units in: (1) general areas of basic biological studies of drug and substance abuse; (2) animal and human studies relevant to the development of an understanding of drug treatment and prevention activities; and (3) epidemiological studies. In addition, a unit to disseminate information to researchers, clinicians and the public will be created.

The current objectives of NIDA are therefore to: (1) collect and analyze data on the nature and extent of drug abuse, while monitoring emergent trends in drug use; (2) sponsor and conduct basic and applied research on drugs and related brain and body phenomena, on the etiology and epidemiology of drug abuse and on prevention and treatment rehabilitation techniques and strategies; (3) disseminate public information and sponsor programs of active discouragement of drug misuse and abuse; (4) disseminate these research findings to all agencies or interested parties involved in drug abuse prevention, treatment and rehabilitation; and (5) upon request, lend assistance to such agencies and individuals in carrying out drug abuse programs.

RECENT ACCOMPLISHMENTS

Basic research represents approximately fifty percent of NIDA's total research program. The long-range goal of basic biomedical research activities is to increase an understanding of the physiological mechanisms of drug tolerance, dependence and addiction. Toward this end studies are supported that focus on the sites and mechanisms of drug use.

Epidemiological research has provided information on the extent and nature of drug use in both the general population as well as selected subgroups. Research support has also been provided in an attempt to determine the biological, psychological and social factors that make persons particularly vulnerable to drug abuse. Prevention related research has been subdivided into (1) the development and evaluation of various drug abuse approaches and (2) the determination of the abuse liability of the various substances.

Drug hazard research has been supported to more clearly define direct biologic hazards, such as genetic and reproductive effects, indirect hazards resulting from effects on sociologic function and psychomotor performance, and long-term consequences resulting from drug use and abuse. Treatment research supported in the past has involved the evaluation of current treatment forms, the efficacy of new therapeutic methods for treating drug abuse, the exploration of promising nonpharmacological modalities, such as psychotherapy and other disciplines in addressing drug abuse, and the development and assessment of innovative programs designed to meet the needs of special populations.

The NIDA research program has made several major contributions to the study of drug and substance abuse in the past several years. A brief description of these consists of the following:

Opiate Receptors and Endogenous Opiate-Like Substances

Over the last several years NIDA-sponsored research was responsible for the identification and isolation of opiate receptors within the central nervous system and the subsequent discovery of endogenous opiate-like substances. This research has sparked vigorous work not only in the area of drug abuse but also in the fields of neurological disease, mental health, cardiac function, and pain and analgesia. Furthermore, these findings provide the first testable hypothesis for a biological basis of addiction, i.e., that addiction may be the result of disorders of the endorphin-enkephalin system which could result in the decreased production of endorphins and enkephalins (as in the diabetes model where the disease results from decreased production of insulin), or reduced responsivity resulting from reduced receptor sensitivity. Tests on these hypotheses are just beginning. The findings of these studies will open new methods for the prevention and treatment of drug abuse and other health problems.

Development of an Ongoing Epidemiological Data Base

Until recently, the epidemiology of drug abuse has been viewed as extremely difficult and uncertain because of the illicit nature of the activity. As a result of extensive surveys and psychological research, techniques have been developed so that trends in this area can be immediately and reliably assessed. This is of great importance because of the extreme variability of drug abuse phenomena compared to other health problems. Some indices in the drug abuse field, e.g., the incidence of PCP abuse, have increased over 3000 percent in a relatively short period. The Institute has developed three ongoing epidemiological data systems for tracking the incidence, prevalence and trends in drug abuse. These include the Drug Abuse Warning Network (DAWN), the National Household Survey, and the High School Survey. The information provided by these surveys is used to determine priorities for research and prevention programs and to alert the States to new drug abuse problems. For example, with information provided by these surveys, NIDA quickly became aware of the rising problem of PCP abuse a few years ago and the recent leveling off and beginning decline in the use of marijuana by teenagers.

Development of New Treatment Agents

The Institute has continued to develop new and more effective drug abuse treatment agents. The most important of these are LAAM, naltrexone, and buprenorphine. LAAM, because it has a longer duration of action than methadone, will require less frequent visits by patients to treatment clinics. It will result in less disruption to the patient's personal life and employment and should be considerably cheaper than methadone maintenance. NIDA has filed a revised IND with FDA which, if favorably reviewed, could result in LAAM being approved for general use by the FDA in fiscal year 1982. Naltrexone has great promise for patients who want to become totally drug free. It has no opiate-like effects and does not produce physical or psychological dependence, yet it nullifies the effect of opiates. Because of its relatively infrequent administration (twice a week), it should also reduce the cost of treatment. Buprenorphine, which is now being clinically tested at the ARC, is a combination agonist/antagonist. Like methadone, it produces alterations in moods and perceptions that are acceptable to addict patients, but unlike methadone and other narcotics, it causes little or no physical dependence and is unlikely to directly cause death. As a substitute for methadone, it would eliminate or reduce the direct toxic deaths associated with methadone therapy as well as block the effects of narcotics. Its advantage over naltrexone is that patients find it more acceptable, which leads us to believe they will continue therapy at a much greater rate.

Clarification of the Addictive Properties of Nicotine

Nicotine has been found to have reinforcing properties similar to those of alkaloids separated from other natural substances such as cocaine and morphine. Nicotine will, for example, be "self-injected" by addicts given access to nicotine intravenously in much the same manner as other abused drugs. Studies of self-administration in animals indicate patterns of responding similar to that observed with other stimulants such as cocaine. Tobacco has been found to involve pharmacologic and psychologic mechanisms similar to those involved in the compulsive use of other substances, which suggests that both the medical and scientific strategy directed at tobacco use can be modeled after those developed to treat and prevent narcotic addiction.

The NAPA Experiment: School-Based Drug Abuse Prevention

Over the past several years the Institute has sponsored a tightly controlled study of several different drug abuse prevention strategies directed at seventh and eighth graders. Among the strategies tested were drug education courses, teacher training, and decision-making courses. The study revealed clear differences in the efficacies of these and other strategies in changing student attitudes about and use of drugs. Of particular importance, it was found that the most effective course was one directed at increasing students' abilities to resist peer pressure to begin or continue drug use combined with information and discussions about drug use. This finding coincides with the results of studies of successful anti-smoking programs. The results of this study will greatly help in the development of more effective and less costly prevention programs.

Drug Paraphernalia

The Institute has completed the only study ever done of the growth of the drug paraphernalia market. The study notes ways in which community groups and State and local legislative bodies have been able to control the availability of drug paraphernalia. The report developed by this study has been widely requested by State legislative bodies and private groups.

Drug Use in Rural Areas

The Institute has conducted a large-scale national investigation of drug use patterns in rural areas. The study found that drug use in rural areas is rapidly increasing and beginning to resemble drug use patterns typically found in urban areas. The report developed by this study is available to State agency officials and may be used in planning the delivery of drug abuse treatment and prevention services.

Treatment Research

An extensive series of studies have begun to reveal which types of treatment are most effective for particular types of individuals with serious drug abuse problems. For example, large numbers of addicts have been found to be clinically depressed and their addiction treatment outcome is significantly improved if their depression is separately but concurrently treated. Certain addicts have been found to do less well as the length of treatment is extended; others show greater improvement the longer they stay in treatment. Depending on the type and severity of the psychopathology, some patients improve more rapidly with structured psychotherapy in addition to counseling. Once we better understand how to predict the success of various combinations of treatment modalities for particular kinds of addicts, we will be able to reduce the cost of treatment by more appropriately assigning treatment regimens.

CONCLUSION

In summary, NIDA, while undergoing an internal structural reorganization, will continue to provide support for research in all major areas of drug abuse. Through such support it is anticipated that a better understanding of the pathophysiology, psychology, epidemiology, and efficacy of treatment will be developed. This in turn will allow the improvement of clinical care to those abusing drugs and permit a greater awareness on both the part of health professionals and the public of the problems associated with drug abuse and its management.

The National Institute on Drug Abuse: Priorities in Funding

Jack Durell, MD, and the Staff
at the National Institute
on Drug Abuse

ABSTRACT. In accomplishing NIDA's twofold mission of understanding the processes underlying drug abuse and searching for new knowledge in preventing, detecting, diagnosing, and treating the problem, the Institute has in place an intramural and extramural research program. The intramural program supports clinical and biomedical research projects which are conducted at the Institute's Addiction Research Center in Baltimore, Maryland. The extramural program supports research conducted by investigators at other institutions.

The extramural research support mechanisms are diverse, but can be divided into two main categories: grants and contracts. Grants are usually unsolicited and the applicant investigator is responsible for developing the ideas, concepts, methods, and approach for a research project. Contracts are solicited, and the awarding institute is responsible for establishing the plans, parameters, and detailed requirements for a project.

NIDA also has two major support mechanisms for talented investigators which are (1) the ADAMHA Research Scientists Development and Research Scientists Program and (2) the ADAMHA Research Service Awards for Individual Fellows. The purpose of these awards is to enable exceptionally talented investigators to engage in long-term research programs related to drug abuse. Interdisciplinary basic and applied research proposals are encouraged from scientists in medical schools, departments of psychiatry, nonmedical academic departments, psychiatric hospitals, biomedical research institutes, and departments of behavioral science.

In accordance with NIDA's organizational structure, basic and applied research is being conducted in the three major areas of preclinical, clinical, and epidemiological. NIDA-supported research

Dr. Durell is Associate Director for Science, National Institute on Drug Abuse, 5600 Fishers Lane, Rockville, Maryland 20857.

in these areas must be clearly related to the etiology, prevalence, prediction, diagnosis, clinical course, treatment, management or prevention of drug abuse or other drug-related health problems or their consequences.

To fully accomplish the described mission of the Institute, NIDA continually searches for the most effective mechanisms for disseminating research findings to the general public, health care professionals, and organizations involved in drug abuse treatment and prevention. The goal is to see federally supported research positively impact on the State and local administered drug abuse treatment and prevention programs.

The basic mission of NIDA is to improve the health of the nation by (1) increasing our understanding of the processes underlying drug abuse and (2) acquiring new knowledge to help prevent, detect, diagnose, and treat disease. NIDA accomplishes this mission by: (1) supporting research in universities, medical schools, hospitals, and research institutions in this country and abroad; (2) conducting research in its own laboratories and clinics; (3) supporting training for promising young researchers; (4) helping to develop and maintain research resources; (5) identifying research findings which can be applied to the care of patients and helping to transfer such advances to the health care system; (6) promoting effective ways to communicate biomedical information to scientists, health practitioners and the public; and (7) developing and recommending policies related to the conduct and support of biomedical research.

In order to achieve these goals, the NIDA relies on its intramural and extramural programs. The intramural programs support clinical and biomedical research projects conducted at the Addiction Research Center, while the extramural programs provide funding for investigators at other institutions.

MECHANISMS OF SUPPORT

The diverse support mechanisms for extramural research are divided into two main categories: grants and contracts. Grants typically support individual research projects and program projects, as well as fellowships, research training programs, and Research Career Development Awards; clinical trials may be funded either by grants or contracts. In general, with grants, the applicant investigator is responsible for developing the ideas, concepts, methods, and approach for a research project; with contracts, however, the awarding institute is responsible for establishing the plans, parameters and detailed requirements for a project. Contracts are solicited through requests for proposals (RFPs), while grants are not usually solicited. In certain circumstances, however, grants are solicited to support areas of special interest to an awarding unit, in which case requests for applications (RFAs) and program announcements are issued. Other distinctions between contracts and grants involve such technical issues as the cost reimbursement and mechanisms for monitoring, the extent of involvement of the sponsoring Institute, and the delivery of the end product.

Grant applications are classified according to type, such as new, competing continuation (renewal), and supplementary applications, and according to activities, such as traditional research projects, conferences, program projects, and fellowships. Contract proposals are classified according to transaction types, such as new, renewal, modification, and continuation of incrementally funded contracts.

Another form of support, called the cooperative agreement, has recently been legislatively mandated. The cooperative agreement, like the grant, is oriented to support or stimulate the recipient's activities, but provides for substantial involvement on the part of the funding agency during the period of performance.

Specific Programs for Individual Investigator Support

The two major supports provided by NIDA for talented investigators are (1) the ADAMHA Research Scientist Development and Research Scientist Program and (2) the ADAMHA Research Service Awards for Individual Fellows. The purpose of the ADAMHA Research Scientist Program is to foster the development of outstanding scientists and to enable them to expand their potential for making important contributions in the fields of alcoholism, drug abuse, or mental health research. This is accomplished by providing several types of awards to enable exceptionally talented investigators to engage essentially full-time on a long-term basis in research, and to enhance their skills and dedication to these areas of research. Awards are made to institutions on behalf of specific outstanding individuals. Applications are encouraged for scientists working in a variety of institutions with research programs related to alcoholism, drug abuse, and mental health—such as medical schools, departments of psychiatry, non-medical academic departments, psychiatric hospitals or hospitals with psychiatric services, biomedical research institutes and departments of behavioral science. Interdisciplinary research proposals are encouraged, and applications for both basic and applied research will be supported.

Awards provided for these programs may support up to $30,000 in basic salary for the individual candidate, fringe benefits, and indirect cost allowance not to exceed 8%, specialized training costs when justified, and limited research costs under certain circumstances.

Research Scientist Development Awards

There are two types of available awards. Level I awards are designed to support individuals with exceptional research potential who need further supervised research experience in a productive scientific environment. The typical applicant is a young scientist just finishing his/her postdoctoral training. Others may be candidates who are adequately prepared in one scientific discipline and desire extensive supervised experience in another discipline, or may desire supervised clinical experience so as to develop a clinical research capacity. In all instances, the hallmark of a Level I application is the need for extensive supervised research experience. Applicants whose background is primarily clinical should be most careful to emphasize their plans for supervised research experience and document their potential for developing into an excellent researcher.

Level II awards are designed to support individuals with excellent preparation in their scientific discipline. They should be capable of designing and conducting excellent independent, original research projects, but need additional research experience in order to realize their potential as outstanding research scientists. Applicants for these awards are typically persons with excellent training and a highly promising research record or those who are successfully completing a Level I award.

Research Scientist Awards

Research Scientist Awards are designed to support exceptional senior investigators in appropriate departments and centers where institutional funds would not be available for support of such investigators in essentially full-time research positions. While most awards at this level represent continuation of support at the developmental levels, it is possible for a senior investigator moving into full-time research or moving to a new institution to start with the Research Scientist Award.

Research Service Awards for Individual Fellows

An Individual National Research Service Award provides support to individuals for predoctoral and postdoctoral research training in specified drug abuse-related areas. ADAMHA is concentrating its funding on postdoctoral research training.

Research fellowships are funded in a wide variety of biomedical, clinical, psychological and behavioral disciplines, including chemistry, biochemistry, physiology, pharmacology, toxicology, genetics, neuroscience, psychology, psychiatry, and social science as they relate to drug abuse. Specific areas of interest for which the training of individual investigators will be supported include: (1) basic processes of brain and behavior as they relate to drug abuse; (2) incidence and prevalence of drug abuse; (3) etiology, description, diagnosis and pathogenesis; (4) treatment research; and (5) public health and prevention research.

Institutional Training Grants and Contracts

The Research Service Awards for Institutional Grants serve a similar purpose to that seen with the individual investigator awards. However, the Institutional Grant allows nonprofit institutions to develop research training opportunities for individuals interested in careers in particular specified drug abuse-related fields.

SCIENTIFIC AREAS ELIGIBLE FOR FUNDING

In regard to the various support mechanisms described above, NIDA is interested in supporting a variety of studies, including:

Epidemiology of Drug Abuse: Studies designed to determine the incidence and prevalence of nonmedical use and abuse of all classes of psychoactive drugs; exploration of the patterns, trends and extent of drug use; studies of drug users and abusers drawn from varied cultural and ethnic backgrounds; studies or demonstration projects on special or high risk populations; development and evaluation of methodologies and statistical techniques to assess the nature and extent of drug use; studies on the natural history of drug abuse; studies of the historical development of drug use and abuse; the use of psychological tests, surveys and other methods to determine the extent of drug use; assessment of the impact of changes in law on the incidence and prevalence of drug abuse; and development of techniques to facilitate the identification of target groups at risk.

Etiology of Drug Abuse: Investigations into biological, psychiatric, psychological factors and environmental conditions as possible causes of drug and substance use and abuse; studies of the pharmacological, biochemical or neurochemical bases of the abuse liability of drugs, inhalants, volatiles or other substances including tobacco; studies of the pharmacological, biochemical and neurochemical bases of the phenomena of drug and substance abuse; studies of personality or behavioral factors which may predispose an individual to abuse drugs; longitudinal research studies which are concerned with factors which may be predictive of subsequent drug abuse; personality factors determining choice of drug abuse as an adaptive mechanism or as a manifestation of psychopathology; studies of familial factors and the influence of peers on the abuse of drugs; studies of small group processes and dynamics associated with the initiation, continuation and termination of drug use; investigations using learning principles involved in the acquisition, maintenance and extinction of drug-seeking behavior; psychometric tests and measurement scales for predicting drug abusing behavior or resistance to drug abuse.

Drug Abuse Treatment: A wide range of studies demonstrating the effectiveness of current and innovative nonpharmacologic treatment methods are considered for funding. Special priority is given to the following areas: (1) development and evaluation of treatment methods that are specifically focused on the needs of child and adolescent drug abusers and those that focus on the family; (2) studies intended to improve the differential diagnosis of drug abusers so that the categories are of greater clinical relevance; (3) well-controlled studies testing the effectiveness of differing counseling or psychotherapeutic approaches, particularly if they are carefully related to specific diagnostic sub-categories; (4) development and preclinical and clinical evaluation of new narcotics and narcotic antagonists and nonaddicting analgesic drugs; (5) evaluation or demonstration of the effectiveness of treatment methods which include synthesis and development of long-acting or depot preparations for sustained drug delivery of treatment agents;

development and demonstration of new pharmacological treatment methods for narcotic addiction, including both antagonist and substitution approaches.

Prevention: Support is given to a wide range of studies focusing on the development, demonstration, and outcome evaluation of approaches to prevention of drug abuse through programs of information, education, early intervention and community resource mobilization and coordination. Projects should focus upon prevention theory development and the testing of strategies designed to prevent or reduce drug use behavior, particularly for individuals at high risk. Particular priority would be given to projects involving peer and cross-age interaction strategies which include drug-specific materials and skill-building training to resist peer pressures; projects involving family-oriented prevention programs and those testing drug abuse prevention interventions applicable in the work setting, with the objective of improving productivity and work safety. Development of new methods for assessing addiction liability and abuse potential of narcotic and nonnarcotic drugs and other substances; development of analgesic drugs of low abuse potential; studies of the abuse potential of prescription drugs and factors leading to abuse; industrial and environmental settings and their relationship to substance abuse, changes in drug abuse law and its enforcement, as well as other control mechanisms as prevention methods.

Adverse Effects and Clinical Pharmacology of Abuse Substances: Adverse biomedical, psychiatric, psychological and behavioral consequences of abused drugs and other substances; clinical pharmacology of opiates, marijuana, and other abused drugs or substances with abuse potential. Animal toxicity studies and evaluation of safety of compounds used in treatment of drug abuse; studies of the effects of abused drugs or substances, including genetic, mutagenic and teratogenic and other adverse effects on prenatal or postnatal development and growth, and of effects on fertility, hormonal balance, development and reproduction. Studies on the effects of the interactions of abused drugs with one another and/or with other abused substances or with therapeutic drugs; studies of the effects of drugs of abuse during disease, advancing age, or other altered physiological states. Behavioral toxicity and potential deleterious effects of single drugs and drug interactions on body organs and systems; studies of psychiatric/psychological complications of drug abuse; effects of drug and substance abuse on behavior and performance, such as driving, learning, memory, school performance and adverse consequences associated with drug abuse, such as crime and delinquency.

Basic Research and Methodological Development: Research on the basic mechanisms of action of abused drugs or substances, including tobacco, and the mechanisms involved in the phenomena of tolerance, dependence, enkephalins, endorphins, and other endogenous substances and their receptors as these relate to the problems of drug abuse and analgesia; studies of the perception of pleasure or pain as these relate to the problem of drug abuse, and studies of analgesia. Studies of the pharmacodynamics, pharmacokinetics, and metabolism of abused drugs or substances and of drugs used to treat narcotic addiction. Studies of the mechanisms by which drugs used to treat narcotic and other drug addictions exert their effects. Fundamental studies on the mechanisms of reinforcement and its biological substrates which may relate to the addiction process; research on abused drugs and other substances which utilize biochemical, pharmacological, neuroendocrine, behavioral, physiochemical or biophysical approaches; development of analytical and synthetic methods for the study of drug metabolites. Studies of naturally occurring sources of substances of abuse, such as cannabis, coca, opium, or papaver species.

Studies supported by NIDA must be clearly related to the etiology, prevalence, prediction, diagnosis, clinical course, treatment, management or prevention of drug abuse or other drug-related health problems, or to consequences of these health problems. Social research studies will not be supported unless they explicitly focus on investigation of the above factors. For example, research on changing social roles or rising crime rates as general social phenomena will not be supported; however, research in these areas which is explicitly focused on the relationship, such as the changing roles of women and the development or treatment of drug abuse, or on the relationship of drug abuse to the occurrence of family violence would be supported by NIDA.

SUMMARY OF RESEARCH PRIORITIES

NIDA's research program, therefore, has two basic goals: (1) to understand the mechanisms which underlie the development and/or perpetuation of dysfunctional drug use and (2) to find the best means of preventing and treating the problem. Although great reliance will be placed on extramural research, efforts will by no means be limited to investigator-initiated research. The Institute's research efforts will be shaped by a number of clear objectives and will include a certain amount of directed research, particularly in the areas of treatment, abuse-liability, drug-supply and quantification, and new drug hazards, such as cocaine and "look-alike" drugs, which require quick response. Some of these areas will be addressed in extramural research projects; others are less suitable or interesting for outside investigators and will instead be the focus of study at the Federal Government's intramural drug abuse research facility, the Addiction Research Center (ARC) in Baltimore. Still other priority areas will be developed through Requests for Proposals.

Through support of both intramural and extramural projects, basic and applied research will be conducted in three major areas—preclinical, clinical and epidemiological.

NIDA will continue to support a broad-based program as indicated in the preceding section. However, because of their important public health significance, certain areas of applied research are particularly encouraged and well-designed studies in these areas will be given special consideration. These areas include:

1. Detailed studies of the effects of commonly abused drugs on cognitive and visualmotor performance measures with particular attention to the time course of these effects.
2. Chronic toxicity studies of commonly abused drugs such as marijuana and cocaine.
3. Studies on risk factors that predispose to progression from casual use to heavy and regular use of drugs of abuse such as cocaine, marijuana and stimulants.
4. Studies that relate the differential effects of varying treatment approaches to well-defined sub-categories of patients or diagnostic groups.
5. The development and evaluation of treatment approaches for adolescent drug abusers, including those approaches emphasizing time-limited cost-effectiveness means of involving the adolescent's family with treatment and/or educative approaches.
6. Studies designed to develop and evaluate strategies for preventing drug abuse in youth—with particular priority on studies utilizing skill-building techniques to teach resistance to peer pressure and studies involving family-based strategies.
7. Studies designed to develop and evaluate techniques for using

the communications media to help in the prevention of drug abuse.

8. Studies designed to determine the clinical relevance of our knowledge of basic mechanism of drug action such as studies on the role of endogenous opioids in the predisposition to and progression of addictive disorders.

The above listing of areas of applied research to be given priority is not meant to exclude a continuing priority in basic research. No biomedical research program could hope to be successful over its long-range without continuing to support advances in basic knowledge. NIDA will continue to support studies on the basic mechanisms involved in the action of drugs of abuse, including studies of receptors and endogenous ligands. Moreover, we wish to encourage such studies for drugs such as marijuana in which little is known about basic mechanisms of action. Finally, NIDA wishes to increase research on the basic brain mechanisms relevant to the behavioral systems involved in drug abuse. Thus, study of the brain mechanisms involved in reinforcement, pleasure and pain, various compulsive behavior and in processes such as tolerance, dependence and withdrawal will be encouraged.

Finally, an essential element of the Institute's overall research strategy will be to explore and implement the most effective mechanisms for disseminating research findings to the general public, health care professionals, and organizations involved in drug abuse treatment and prevention. Current efforts, such as colloquia, symposia, workshops and publications, will be continued and expanded, and new means identified in order to see that research carried on at the Federal level has the greatest and swiftest possible impact on those planning and directing drug abuse treatment and prevention programs at the State and local level.

The Application Processes at the National Institute on Drug Abuse and the National Institute on Alcohol Abuse and Alcoholism

Jack Durell, MD, and the Staff
at the National Institute on Drug Abuse
and the National Institute on Alcohol
Abuse and Alcoholism

ABSTRACT. NIDA and NIAAA support individual and institutional research efforts through several different kinds of grants. Those most commonly awarded include: Individual Research Grants; Individual postdoctoral National Research Service Awards; Institutional National Research Service Awards; Research Career Development Awards; and New Investigator Research Awards. Grants are also made for research demonstration and dissemination projects, for program projects, and for conferences.

Grant applications are submitted to the Division of Research Grants at NIH, then assigned to the appropriate Institute by the ADAMHA Grants Review and Referral Office. Each application receives two sequential levels of review. The first level involves panels of experts, known as Scientific Review Groups or Initial Review Groups, who evaluate the scientific and technical merit of each grant proposal. The second level of review is by NIDA's or NIAAA's National Advisory Council, who look also at the application's relevance to the Institute's programs and priorities. Overall, applications are evaluated on the basis of: scientific significance and originality; appropriateness and adequacy of the research approach and methodology; qualifications and experience of the researchers; availability of resources; and reasonable nature of project's budget and time frame.

After an application has been approved through the dual review process, it is considered for funding. An application that has been

Dr. Durell is Associate Director for Science, National Institute on Drug Abuse, 5600 Fishers Lane, Rockville, Maryland 20857.

approved is not automatically funded; this depends on the award criteria of each program and on total funds available. If an application has been approved and a decision to fund it made, an award statement is issued by the Institute's Grants Management Office.

INTRODUCTION

The Alcohol, Drug Abuse and Mental Health Administration (ADAMHA), by means of various grant mechanisms and contracts, solicits and supports research activities pertinent to each of its three Institutes.* The application process and policies described herein for the National Institute on Drug Abuse (NIDA) and the National Institute on Alcohol Abuse and Alcoholism (NIAAA) are ADAMHA-wide, and, in great part, follow policies and procedures set by the Public Health Service (PHS); therefore, this paper will describe the process followed by all three Institutes, with any minor differences and exceptions noted.

KINDS OF SUPPORT

Grant applications are solicited from the field, primarily from researchers in institutions of higher education. The general types of grants currently supported by NIAAA and NIDA include: 1) regular research grants; 2) program projects; 3) regular and clinical research centers; 4) cooperative agreements; 5) the National Research Service Award program, which includes research fellowships and institutional grants; 6) small grants; 7) research scientist development awards; 8) new investigator research awards; and 9) conference grants.

SPECIFIC TYPES OF RESEARCH
AND RESEARCH TRAINING GRANTS

Applications can be submitted for support through the specific grant programs listed below.

Individual Research Grants. Applications for this type of award

---

*Descriptions of these mechanisms are available in NIH Manual Issurance 4101, *Activity Codes, Organizational Codes, and Definitions Used in Extramural Programs,* October 1982.

are those most often reviewed in the committee meetings of NIDA's and NIAAA's Initial Review Groups (IRGs). This program is designed to support the research efforts of individual scientists on discrete, circumscribed projects of their choosing.

Individual Postdoctoral National Research Service Awards (F32). This award is presented to an individual who is sponsored by an established investigator for a period of up to 3 years. The F32 provides newly graduated scientists and physicians with additional research training to broaden their scientific skills and research potential in specific health-related areas. Fellowship applications are not routinely reviewed by Council.

Research Demonstration and Dissemination Projects. These grants, awarded by NIDA, support health service activities and foster the spread of existing knowledge to control specific diseases.

The Institutional National Research Service Award (T-32). This institutional fellowship is slightly different from the F32. The objectives are similar, but the T-32s are awarded to institutions, which then select the particular individuals to be trained.

The Research Science Development Awards (ADAMHA). These awards support scientists who are committed to research, but in need of additional experience.

The New Investigator Research Award. This program is designed to encourage new investigators, including those who have interrupted early promising careers in basic or clinical science disciplines to develop their research interests and capabilities in biomedical and behavioral research. To help bridge the transition from training status to that of established investigator, this special grant supported program provides research grant funds for relatively inexperienced investigators with meritorious research ideas.

Program Project Grants (PO1). These grants support broadly based, multidisciplinary research efforts with a well-defined central research focus or objective. This type of application consists of a number of interrelated projects that contribute to the program objective. The responsibility for leadership of the program resides with the principal investigator or program director who must possess demonstrated scientific and administrative competence. Each of the subprojects is led by an established investigator.

Conference Grants. These are awarded to established scientists for support of conferences or workshops on specific topics of current scientific or clinical interest.

Applications from Foreign Institutions may be reviewed by Study

Sections, either under one of the programs mentioned above or under a program (PL480) administered by the Fogarty International Center. Foreign applicants are not eligible for all types of grants mentioned above.

GENERAL REVIEW CRITERIA

The Initial Review Group (IRG) provides an evaluation of the merit of each application. The principal criteria for the initial review of applications for project grants include: 1) scientific, technical, or medical significance and originality of the proposed research; 2) appropriateness and adequacy of the experimental approach and methodology to be used; 3) qualifications and experience of the principal investigator and staff in the area of the research; 4) availability of research facilities and other resources; and 5) reasonableness of the proposed budget and duration.

Where an application involves activities which could have an adverse effect upon humans, animals, or the environment, the adequacy of the proposed means for protecting against or minimizing such effects are also evaluated.

The principal criteria for the review of applications for individual follow-up awards: 1) adequacy and appropriateness of the candidate's training; 2) significance and originality of the candidate's previous research experience and proposed research; 3) candidate's potential for becoming an independent investigator; 4) the relationship of the training of the candidate's future objectives; and 5) the institutional commitment to fostering the candidate's research career, as reflected in the extent to which the candidate will be relieved of other academic responsibilities to provide additional time for research, and the provision of adequate laboratory facilities, equipment, and opportunities for critical professional interaction with colleagues. Depending on the specific kind of award involved, greater emphasis is placed on specific criteria.

RECEIPT AND ASSIGNMENT OF APPLICATIONS

Role of NIH's Division of Research Grants (DRG)

The earliest stage in the processing of competing grant applications involves the sending of a completed grant application by the applicant to a central receipt point. ADAMHA makes use of a centralized system in collaboration with NIH. Specifically, NIH's Division of Research Grants (DRG) has been designated as the official point for receipt, initial referral, collection of administrative data, and duplication and distribution of all ADAMHA competing grant applications. DRG also provides receipt and processing services for non-competing continuation and non-competing supplemental applications. The key participants in the central receipt, assignment and initial processing of competing applications include DRG staff such as the DRG Referral Officers, who initially screen applications, and the ADAMHA Grants Review and Referral Officer (GRRO), who makes a determination as to relevance and acceptability of a grant application, and assigns each accepted application to the appropriate Institute and Initial Review Group (IRG). The GRRO assigns grant applications on the basis of a set of referral guidelines which have been provided by both Institute program and review staff to the GRRO. The GRRO also preliminarily assigns to an Institute program unit which would be responsible for funding the application, but Institute program staff have the final responsibility for ensuring the assignment is accurate; requests for any changes or transfers are sent to the Institute's Review Director.

Following assignment by the ADAMHA GRRO, DRG duplicates and distributes copies of the applications to the appropriate Executive Secretary, who is responsible for the management and coordination of the assigned IRG. DRG also sends the original and copies to the Institute's Grants Management Branch. Also DRG collects basic administrative data from applications and inputs them into a computerized system which serves as a central source of information on applications and grants. This system is also used to generate other documents and reports used in the review and award processes.

Receipt Dates and Review Cycles

A general schedule has been developed for all PHS applications (incorporating NIAAA and NIDA) that are centrally received by DRG, NIH. The purpose of this schedule is to enable involved staff to handle application receipt, assignment, and review in an orderly and efficient manner, with maximum prior notice to applicants for preparing applications.

ADAMHA program announcements may be sent to the field with a special receipt deadline, but the major ongoing grant programs of ADAMHA follow the receipt schedule outlined in Table 1.

TABLE 1

RECEIPT AND ASSIGNMENT OF APPLICATIONS

RECEIPT DATE[1]	IRG MEETING	COUNCIL MEETING
February 1[2] March 1[3]	June	September - October (3rd and 4th weeks of September/1st and 2nd weeks of October)
June 1[2] July 1[3]	October - November (2nd to 4th week of October/1st to 3rd week of November)	January - February (4th week of January/ 1st week of February)
October 1[2] November 1[3]	February - March (2nd to 4th week of February/1st to 3rd week of March)	May (3rd and 4th weeks of May)

[1]Small grant applications may be submitted any time during the year, and will be reviewed five times a year.

[2]Receipt dates for competing continuation applications for research grants; new and competing and continuation applications for Research Scientist Development Awards; and new and competing continuation applications for individual and institutional National Research Service Awards.

[3]Receipt dates for new and supplemental research grants.

THE GRANTS DUAL REVIEW SYSTEM

The magnitude, diversity, and complexity of their research missions, as well as their pursuit of excellence, necessitates that both NIDA and NIAAA draw for assistance on the national pool of scientists actively engaged in research to serve as reviewers. These scientists assist by advising on the selection of the most meritorious and most promising research projects for support.

The grants peer review system used by the NIDA and NIAAA (as well as other ADAMHA/NIH Institutes) is referred to as the "dual review system," and is based on two sequential levels of review for each grant application. Both levels are statutorily mandated. The first level involves panels of experts established according to scientific disciplines or medical specialty areas, whose primary function is to evaluate the scientific and technical merit of grant applications. These panels are referred to as scientific review groups (SRGs) or Study Sections or initial review groups (IRGs).

The second level of review is by National Advisory Councils, which are composed of both scientific and lay representatives noted for their expertise, interest, or leadership in the fields of alcohol and drug abuse. Council recommendations are based not only on consideration of scientific and technical merit as judged by an IRG, but also on the relevance of a grant application to an Institute's programs and priorities.

The dual review system therefore separates the scientific assessment of proposed projects from policy decisions about scientific areas to be supported and the level of resources to be allocated. This permits a more objective evaluation than would result from a single level of review. This system provides the responsible NIDA and NIAAA officials with the best available advice about scientific as well as societal values and needs.

Staff Responsibilities

The initial review process is managed by a central office in each Institute. This office is organizationally separate from and operates independently of the Institute's program divisions. The Director of each Institute's review office is responsible for establishing Institute review policies and procedures, and for managing all aspects of the peer (IRG) review process. The Executive Secretaries of each IRG and their staffs are part of this review office.

The Executive Secretary, assisted by staff, has the most significant responsibilities for grant applications prior to, during, and following IRG review. This person is a professional health scientist administrator with experience in the area of IRG management, and is responsible for assuring that each application assigned for review by the IRG receives appropriate technical and fair review according to established policies and procedures, keeps adequate records of the IRG's recommendations and supporting reasons, and ensures that conflict-of-interest situations are avoided. Typically IRG members are appointed for 4-year terms. The nomination and review process for IRG member selection is initiated by the Executive Secretary. Factors considered in selection are professional competence, and the particular balance of expertise, minorities and women, and geographic distribution needed at that time. IRGs are composed almost exclusively of non-Federal employees, and only one person from a particular institution may serve at one time.

IRG Meetings

Depending on the number of applications being reviewed, the IRG meetings are held for 2-4 days three times a year. After an initial "open" (to the public) session where review procedures, legislative and program development, and other factors impacting on the review process are discussed, the meeting is closed to the public for the review of grant applications, i.e., only members of the IRG and authorized Federal personnel may attend. The Chairman of the IRG conducts the review.[1] Primary, and at least secondary review evaluations for each grant application are presented by the designated reviewers, then site visit reports and outside opinions, if any, are read. Discussion by the IRG members follows. IRG is expected to provide a comprehensive assessment of the scientific and technical merit (quality) of each application (Table 2) and to develop a justification for its recommendation, which is as specific as possible. No IRG member may review an application or be present during discussion and voting on applications where he/she has a real or apparent conflict of interest. After discussion by the IRG, a recommendation for action is made on each application. Possible recommendations include: 1) approval, sometimes with minor changes, such as amount or length of support; 2) disapproval, because of unmet review criteria or hazardous or unethical procedures, but *never* on the basis of lack of program relevance; and, 3) deferred in order to obtain additional information through a site visit or written request.

TABLE 2

COMPONENTS OF PEER REVIEW

Project Plan

Are the goals/aims of the proposed project logical, reasonable, and feasible in light of the current state-of-the-art/field? What is the significance of the proposed project to the state-of-the-art or needs of the field? Are the general approach, organization of the tasks, experiences or services, and the specific methods, procedures, services or training appropriate to the proposed goals? Are they feasible? Are there appropriate plans and procedures for periodically assessing progress and accomplishments? Is the proposed work innovative, is it likely to result in new data or concepts, or to confirm existing ones?

Investigators/Program Staff

Do the training, experience, and competence of the principal investigator/program director qualify him or her highly for the proposed work? Will other individuals involved in the project, particularly key personnel, be capable and highly qualified to carry out the proposed goals and activities of the project?

Project Participants

Are appropriate criteria and procedures specified for the selection involved, are procedures adequate to protect their rights and welfare?

Resources and Environment

Are the facilities and environment suitable for carrying out the project in the proposed manner? Are necessary facilities available and accessible? Are there any unique aspects of the facilities or environment which are relevant to proposed activities? Is there sufficient support (in terms of resources and commitment) from the sponsoring institution (including relevant departments, offices, or other parts of the organization) and any cooperating organizations?

Budget

Is the budget realistic in terms of the goals/aims and specific elements of the project plan? Are all items justified in terms of the activities proposed? Is the proposed project period appropriate to the proposed goals?

If a recommendation is made for approval, an application is then assigned a priority rating, utilizing a ranking system from 1 to 5, based on an assessment on how well the application compares with other applications. Each IRG member's individual ratings are added, averaged and multiplied by 100 to provide a 3-digit rating called a priority score. Such scores (on applications receiving a final recommendation for approval by the Institute's Advisory Council, the final review in the dual review process) serve as a major criterion used in arriving at a decision then made by authorized Institute officials as to whether a grant will be funded. All application materials, reviewers' comments, IRG proceedings and recommendations are treated confidentially. Only through Freedom of Information or Privacy Act requests can materials be released, and then only through established procedures followed by authorized Institute personnel.

Follow-up Procedures

Following the IRG meeting, the Executive Secretary prepares a Summary Statement[2] (often referred to as a "pink sheet" because of being printed on pink paper) for each application reviewed which summarizes the substantive considerations leading the IRG's recommendation on the application, including specific supporting reasons. The Executive Secretary also uses as source documents written critiques of at least two reviewers assigned to evaluate the application, outside opinions, a site visit report, if applicable, and comments made by IRG members during the discussion period at the meeting. The Summary Statement is then transmitted to the National Advisory Council at its next scheduled meeting and serves as the primary document utilized in the final review of applications. In addition, it serves as the primary document by which Institute Officials make decisions on funding applications recommended for approval by Council, and as the official record of the IRG review of that application.

National Advisory Council Review

The National Advisory Council of each Institute provides the second, final level of independent review in the overall review process known as dual review. Through its review of grant applications, each Council provides oversight of the IRG review process and presents a crucial element of public advice on the expenditure of Federal funds. The review also assists the Council in its other major function, i.e., providing advice on Institute policies and programs. Each Institute Director is responsible for establishing policies and procedures for programs and review staffs' responsibilities in presenting applications to the National Advisory Council for review.

Council Composition

According to ADAMHA policy, and in many cases also by law, each Institute's National Advisory Council must review and make a recommendation on each application for competing support in a discretionary grant program.* Each Institute's Council is established by law. The Council membership includes the Institute Director, serving as Chairman, ex-officio members from the Department of Defense and the Veteran's Administration, and 12 members appointed by the Secretary, DHHS. Six of the members are leading medical or scientific authorities in the alcohol or drug abuse fields and six are laymen or public members, with special interests and backgrounds in the areas of the Institutes' programs.

Council Meetings

Applications typically are presented to each Council for their review at three meetings during each year. The particular Council meeting to which an application is assigned for review is determined in accordance with an established schedule (Table 1) included in the announcement for the grant program under which the application is accepted. Because of the large number of applications reviewed, Council members discuss in depth only a limited number of applications, utilizing as their main source document for review the Summary Statements prepared previously by the Executive Secretary of the IRG, based on the initial review. An application which is discussed separately may be voted upon individually at the initiative of the Council, or may be included in the "en bloc" voting, where most applications are considered and recommendations made in groups according to each Institute's organizational program structure.

While the Council's recommendations on grant applications are purely advisory, the approvals or disapprovals they recommend are final decisions, and not appealable. Of course, an applicant may resubmit a revised application through the channels and procedures already discussed. The Council bases its recommendations on grant applications mainly on the appropriateness of the initial (IRG) review for scientific/technical merit and occasionally on policy considerations.

The possible recommendations for action by Council are: 1) concurrence with the Initial Review group; 2) nonconcurrence with the

---

*National Research Service Award research fellowships are an exception to this and do not require Council review. They may be reviewed secondarily by a group consisting of one or two staff persons from each Division, whose function is to report to the Institute Director on many issues of importance in fellowships, such as policy considerations, style, and clarity.

Initial Review Group; and 3) deferral for another review. In the overwhelming percentage of cases, the Council concurs with the IRG recommendations for approval or disapproval, the amount and number of years of support and priority score. In the small number of cases where the Council votes to change the IRG's recommendations, there are specific procedures to be followed.[3]

FUNDING PROCESS

After an application has been approved through the dual review process, it is then considered for funding. An application that has been approved is *not* automatically funded. Only authorized officials of each Institute may make award decisions; they are made on the basis of not only IRG and Council recommendations, but on the award criteria established for each program. Generally the priority score and IRG critique included in the Summary Statement are the primary, though not the only, criteria for funding decisions. Other elements such as relevance of the goals of the proposed project to the mission of the Institute's awarding unit and program, program balance, possible duplication of overlapping support from other agencies, and availability of funds also are considered in the funding decision.

NOTIFICATION TO PRIMARY INVESTIGATOR

Within 30 days of Council action a copy of the Summary Statement for each grant application reviewed by each Institute's National Advisory Council is routinely sent to the principal investigator named in the application. Feedback on the quality of the application is thus provided to the grant application. If an application has been approved and a decision to fund an award has been made, an award statement is issued by the Institute's Grants Management Office.

REFERENCES

1. ADAMHA Orientation Handbook for Members of Initial Review Groups, May 1981.
2. National Institute on Drug Abuse Division of Research Guide for Preparation of Summary Statements - "Pink Sheets" (unpublished).
3. ADAMHA Handbook on Review of Grant Applications, June 1981.

SELECTIVE GUIDE
TO CURRENT REFERENCE SOURCES
ON TOPICS DISCUSSED
IN THIS ISSUE

Grantsmanship, Granting Agencies
and Future Prospects
for Grant Support

James E. Raper, Jr.
Janet L. Cowen
Doris A. Jaeger
Harriet R. Meiss

Each issue of *Advances in Alcohol and Substance Abuse* features a section offering suggestions for locating further information on that issue's theme. In this issue, our intent is to guide readers to selected sources of current information on grantsmanship, granting agencies, and future prospects for grant support.

Some reference sources utilize designated terminology (controlled vocabularies) which must be used to find material on topics of interest. For these we shall indicate a sample of available search terms so that the reader can access suitable sources for his/her pur-

The authors are affiliated with the Gustave L. & Janet W. Levy Library, The Mount Sinai Medical Center of New York, One Gustave L. Levy Place, New York, NY 10029. The authors acknowledge with appreciation the assistance of Ms. Frances Caldararo in the preparation of this manuscript.

poses. Other reference tools use keywords or free-text terms (generally from the title of the document or agency listed). In searching the latter, the user should look under synonyms for the concept in question.

Readers are encouraged to consult with their librarians for further assistance before undertaking research on a topic.

Suggestions regarding the content and organization of this section will be welcomed.

A. SOURCES OF INFORMATION ON GRANTSMANSHIP

1. INDEXING AND ABSTRACTING SOURCES. Publisher, start date, and frequency of publication are noted.

Index Medicus (including *Bibliography of Medical Reviews*). Bethesda, MD, National Library of Medicine, 1960- , monthly.
  See: *MeSH* terms, such as Financing, Government; Foundations; Research Support; Training Support.
Science Citation Index. Philadelphia, Institute for Scientific Information, 1961- , bimonthly.
  See: Permuterm Subject Index (permuted title words).
  See: Citation Index (references from bibliographies of items indexed).

2. ON-LINE BIBLIOGRAPHIC DATA BASES. Listed alphabetically in Section D.

3. BOOKS.

Books in Print. New York, R.R. Bowker Co., annual.
  See: Subject headings, such as Grants-in-aid; Research Grants; Subsidies.
National Library of Medicine Current Catalog. Bethesda, MD, National Library of Medicine, 1965- , quarterly with annual and quinquennial cumulations.
  See: *MeSH* terms as noted in Section A.1 under *Index Medicus.*

4. U.S. GOVERNMENT PUBLICATIONS.

Monthly Catalog of United States Government Publications. Washington, DC, U.S. Government Printing Office, 1895- , monthly with annual cumulations.

See: Listings of agencies, such as Alcohol, Drug Abuse and Mental Health Administration (ADAMHA); National Institute of Mental Health (NIMH); National Institute on Drug Abuse (NIDA); and National Institute on Alcohol Abuse and Alcoholism (NIAAA).

See: Keyword title index.

See: Subject headings, such as Alcoholism; Appropriations and Expenditures; Medical Research; United States, Finance.

5. SPECIALIZED INFORMATION CENTERS.

The Foundation Center.

The Foundation Center, organized in 1956 by a small group of New York City foundations and corporations, has developed into an international service organization assisting grantseekers in selecting from nearly 22,000 active foundations which may be interested in their projects. This objective is met by publishing reference books on foundations and foundation grants and disseminating information on foundations through nationwide public service and educational programs.

In addition to the publications annotated in Section B, The Foundation Center also publishes other reference sources. *COMSEARCH Printouts,* an annual series of computer-generated printouts, provides subject access (e.g., #39—Alcohol and Drug Abuse) and geographic access to *The Foundation Grants Index.* Foundation access is also available through *COMSEARCH Special Topics* which lists foundations by categories, such as asset size, annual grant totals, and company-sponsored foundations. *COMSEARCH Broad Topics* is a series of eleven books covering recent foundation grants in broad subject areas, including *Hospitals and Medical Care Programs* (annual). *Foundation Fundamentals* (1981) is a step-by-step guide for grantseekers.

The Center's public service and educational programs operate through its four main libraries listed below and through an international network of 105 cooperating library collections in all fifty states, Canada, Mexico, Puerto Rico, and the Virgin Islands.

The two "Principal" libraries in New York and Washington, DC contain IRS returns for all foundations in the United States, a complete set of published foundation reports and newsletters, all Foundation Center publications, and large collections of information on foundations, grants, philanthropy and not-for-profit management.

The "Field Office" libraries in Cleveland and San Francisco contain IRS returns for all foundations in the Mid-West and West respectively, as well as extensive collections. These libraries, which are open to the public, also offer weekly orientations and reference services provided by librarians skilled in this special field.

The 105 cooperating collections are housed in larger libraries, open to the public, and administered by each parent library. These contain IRS records for all foundations within their own state, a core collection of Foundation Center publications, and additional reference materials for grantseekers.

The Foundation Center's Associate Program is a fee-based service designed to meet the special requirements of those involved in grantseeking on an ongoing basis. Services offered include: telephone reference service (not otherwise available) and customized computer searches.

A series of seminars and workshops on grantseeking is offered throughout the United States. These low cost educational programs aim at raising the level of information available on funding sources and have been made possible through grants from private sources.

For further information on The Foundation Center, or to locate the nearest cooperating collection, contact the nearest principal library or call (800) 424-9836.

Principal Libraries:

The Foundation Center
888 Seventh Avenue
New York, New York 10106

The Foundation Center
1001 Connecticut Avenue, NW
Washington, DC 20036

Field Offices:

The Foundation Center
Kent H. Smith Library
739 National City Bank Building
629 Euclid Avenue
Cleveland, Ohio 44114

The Foundation Center
312 Sutter Street
San Francisco, California 94108

The Grantsmanship Center (1031 South Grand Ave., Los Angeles, California 90015).

The Center is a not-for-profit training institution offering workshops and seminars throughout the United States on grantsmanship, program management, and fundraising. For information and ˙calendar of upcoming events, call (213) 749-4721 or (800) 421-9512 (outside California).

For additional listings of specialized information centers, see *Directory of Special Libraries and Information Centers*. 6th ed. Detroit, Gale Research Co., 1981.
  See: Subject headings, such as Foundations; Fund Raising; Philanthropy.

B. SOURCES OF INFORMATION ON AGENCIES PROVIDING GRANT SUPPORT.

Annual Register of Grant Support. Chicago, Marquis Who's Who, annual.
  Identifies sources of grant support programs of government agencies, public and private foundations, corporations, community trusts, and professional associations.
Catalog of Federal Domestic Assistance (CFDA). Washington, DC, U.S. Government Printing Office, annual.
  Prepared by the Executive Office of the President, Office of Management and Budget. Provides information on federal government programs.
Commerce Business Daily. Chicago, U.S. Department of Commerce, issued Monday to Friday.
  Gives announcements of Requests for Proposals (RFPs) that are available to organizations.
COMSEARCH. See Section A.5 under The Foundation Center.
Corporation Foundation Profiles. Rev. ed. New York, The Foundation Center, 1981, irregular.
  Analyzes over 200 of the largest company-sponsored foundations.
Directory of Research Grants. Phoenix, AZ, Oryx Press, annual, updated between editions by *Faculty Alert Bulletin* and quarterly supplements.
  Details funding opportunities from a variety of sources.
Foundation Directory. 8th ed. New York, The Foundation Center, 1981, biennial, updated between editions by *Foundation Directory Supplement.*

Describes over 3,000 foundations whose assets exceed $1,000,000 or whose annual grants total $100,000 or more.

The Foundation Grants Index. New York, The Foundation Center, annual. Lists grants of $5000 or more awarded by private foundations.

The Foundation Grants Index Bimonthly. New York, The Foundation Center, 1983- , bimonthly, cumulates to form *The Foundation Grants Index.*

Includes new grants reported to The Foundation Center by nearly 500 major foundations.

Foundation Grants to Individuals. New York, The Foundation Center, 1982, biennial. '

Describes nearly 1000 foundations offering grants to individuals.

Guide to Research Support. Washington, DC, The American Psychological Association, 1981.

Identifies federal sources of funding for behavioral science research.

National Data Book. New York, The Foundation Center, annual. Lists, with brief descriptions, all currently active grantmaking foundations in the U.S. as identified by IRS records.

NIH Guide for Grants and Contracts and its supplements. Washington, DC, U.S. Government Printing Office, irregular.

Announces opportunities, requirements, and changes in grants and contracts of the National Institutes of Health.

Research Awards Index. Bethesda, MD, National Institutes of Health, Division of Research Grants, annual.

Provides information on health research currently conducted by non-federal institutions and supported by the health agencies of the Department of Health and Human Services.

C. SOURCES OF INFORMATION USEFUL IN DETERMINING FUTURE PROSPECTS FOR GRANT SUPPORT.

Drug Research Reports (The Blue Sheet). Washington, DC, Drug Research Reports, 1957- , weekly.

Reports congressional and executive news in the health field. Includes RFPs and grants and contracts awarded by agencies such as NIH and ADAMHA.

Foundation News: The Magazine of Philanthropy. New York, Council on Foundations, 1960- , bimonthly.

Provides current information on projects funded by foundations.

Includes news and features dealing with all areas of philanthropy.

Federal Register. Washington, DC, U.S. Government Printing Office, 1936- , issued Monday to Friday.

Provides information suggesting directions of new grant support and reports changes in current support of federal agencies.

Grants Magazine: The Journal of Sponsored Research. New York, Plenum Press, 1978- , quarterly.

Serves the grantseeking and grantmaking public. Articles deal with government, foundation, and corporation grants as well as grantsmanship.

Washington Report on Medicine & Health. Washington, DC, McGraw-Hill, 1968- , weekly.

Publishes announcements of legislation before Congress pertaining to health programs.

D. ON-LINE BIBLIOGRAPHIC DATA BASES. Examples of search entry points are noted for selected data bases. Consult a librarian who is a computer search analyst for assistance in formulating a search strategy.

CATLINE. Machine-readable version of *National Library of Medicine Current Catalog.*

Use: *MeSH* terms as noted in Section A.1 under *Index Medicus.*

CIS/INDEX. Machine-readable version of *Index to Publications of the United States Congress* (Congressional Information Service).

Provides current access to working papers published by House, Senate and joint committees in the form of hearings, prints, reports, and special publications.

Use: Subject descriptors, such as Alcoholism; Alcohol, Drug Abuse, and Mental Health Administration; Drug Abuse and Treatment; Federal Aid to Medicine; Government Spending; Health Research Act; Medical Research; Research and Development Grants and Contracts.

COMMERCE BUSINESS DAILY. Print counterpart is described in Section B.

Use: Single-term subject descriptors to retrieve information on such topics as contract awards, RFPs, and sponsoring agencies.

DRUG INFO/ALCOHOL USE/ABUSE. Produced by the Hazelden Foundation and the Drug Information Service Center, both in Minnesota, this has no print counterpart.

Use: Title words, such as Appropriations; Funding, Grants; Grantsmanship.

FEDREG, or *FEDERAL REGISTER ABSTRACTS.* Machine-readable version of *Federal Register,* which is described in Section C.

FOUNDATION DIRECTORY. Print counterpart is described in Section B. Broad subject descriptors, such as Medicine, may be combined with single terms representing research interest, donor, geographic area, foundation name, and other significant options.

FOUNDATIONS GRANTS INDEX. Print counterpart is described in Section B.

Use: Keywords.

GPO MONTHLY CATALOG; GPO; GPOM. Machine-readable version of *Monthly Catalog of United States Government Publications.*

Use: Search entry points as noted in Section A.4.

GRANTS. Produced by Oryx Press, Phoenix, AZ. *Directory of Research Grants* (Section B) and other publications of its Grant Information System are contained in this data base, which is the source to more than 1500 grant programs available through government and non-government funding agencies.

Use: General subject descriptors, such as Alcoholism; Drug Abuse.

Use: Keywords.

MEDLINE. Produced by the National Library of Medicine. Contains references from *Index Medicus.*

Use: *MeSH* terms as noted in Section A.1 under *Index Medicus.*

Use: Keywords.

Note: In addition to retrieving articles about grantsmanship and funding policy, it is possible to identify research that has been funded by government or non-government agencies by combining terms representing an area of research with the following subject headings: Support, Non-U.S. Gov't; Support, U.S. Gov't, Non-P.H.S; Support, U.S. Gov't, P.H.S. To identify the specific funding agency, it is necessary to refer to the cited paper.

NATIONAL FOUNDATIONS. Machine-readable version of *National Data Book,* which is described in Section B.

Use: Keywords.

NTIS. Produced by the National Technical Information Service of the U.S. Dept. of Commerce, this data base has no print equivalent. Covers U.S. government-sponsored research and development from over 200 federal agencies.

Use: Keywords.

Use: Subject headings, such as Alcoholism; Allocations; Federal Budgets; Grants.

PHARMACEUTICAL NEWS INDEX. Produced by Data Courier, Inc., this data base contains records from *SCRIP World Pharmaceutical News, FDC Reports (The Pink Sheet), Drug Research Reports (The Blue Sheet),* and other printed publications. Provides current information on such topics as government legislation, regulations, court action, RFPs, and research grant applications.

Use: Single-term subject descriptors.

Use: Keywords from titles.

SCI SEARCH. Machine-readable version of *Science Citation Index.*

Use: Keywords from titles.

SSIE CURRENT RESEARCH. Produced by the Smithsonian Science Information Exchange, this data base has no print counterpart. Reports both government and privately-funded research projects, either currently in progress or completed within the last two years.

Use: Keywords.

Use: SSIE subject descriptors, such as Alcoholism and Alcohol Abuse; Drug Addiction and Abuse.

Note: This data base has transferred ownership from the Smithsonian Science Information Exchange to the National Technical Information Service; new records have not been added since February 1982.